Topical Steroids in Gastroenterology and Hepatology

Topical Steroids in Gastroenterology and Hepatology

Edited by

A. Dignass
*Medizinische Klinik mit Schwerpunkt
Hepatologie und Gastroenterologie
Campus Virchow-Klinikum des
Universitätsklinikums Charité
D-13353 Berlin, Germany*

H.J. Buhr
*Universitätsklinikum Benjamin Franklin
der Freien Universität Berlin
Hindenburgdamm 30
D-12203 Berlin, Germany*

V. Gross
*Innere Medizin II
Klinikum St. Marien Amberg
D-92224 Amberg
Germany*

O.F.W. James
*University of Newcastle
The Medical School
Centre for Liver Research
Newcastle upon Tyne, NE2 4HH
United Kingdom*

*Proceedings of the Falk Workshop (New Findings on Pathogenesis and Progress
in Management of Inflammatory Bowel Diseases, Part III) held in Berlin,
Germany, June 14, 2003*

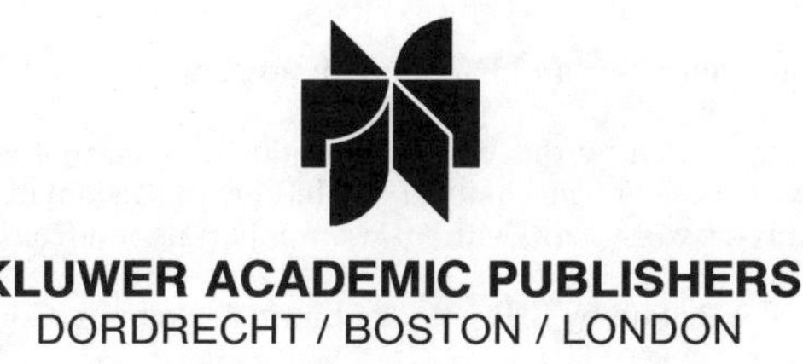

KLUWER ACADEMIC PUBLISHERS
DORDRECHT / BOSTON / LONDON

Library of Congress Cataloging-in-Publication Data is available.

ISBN 0-7923-8789-9

Published by Kluwer Academic Publishers BV,
PO Box 17, 3300 AA Dordrecht, The Netherlands

Sold and distributed in North, Central and South America
by Kluwer Academic Publishers, PO Box 358,
Accord Station, Hingham, MA 02018-0358, USA

In all other countries, sold and distributed
by Kluwer Academic Publishers, Distribution Center,
PO Box 322, 3300 AH Dordrecht, The Netherlands

Printed on acid-free paper

Printed and bound in Great Britain by MPG Books Limited, Bodmin, Cornwall.

Contents

Section III: POTENTIAL USE OF BUDESONIDE AFTER SURGICAL INTERVENTIONS AND IN PATIENTS WITH ONCOLOGICAL COMPLICATIONS

Section IV: POTENTIAL USE OF BUDESONIDE IN HEPATOLOGY

List of principal contributors

F Baert
H Hart Ziekenhuis
Gastroenterologie
Wilgenstraat 2
B-8800 Roeselare
Belgium

H Bertz
Innere Medizin I
Universitätsklinikum Freiburg
Hugstetter Str. 55
D-79106 Freiburg
Germany

HJ Buhr
Chirurgie I
Universitatsklinikum Benjamin
  Franklin der Freien Universitäts
  Berlin
Hindenburgdamm 30
D-12203 Berlin
Germany

A Dignass
Medizinische Klinik mit Schwerpunkt
  Hepatologie und
  Gastroenterologie
Campus Virchow-Klinikum des
  Universitätsklinikums Charité
Augustenburger Platz 1
D-13353 Berlin
Germany

K-W Ecker
Klinik für Allgemeine, Viszerale und
  Gefässchirurgie
Müritz-Klinikum
Weinbergstrasse 19
D-17192 Waren (Müritz)
Germany

S Elad
Hospital Oral Medicine Department
Hadassah University Hospital
Ein Kerem
POB 12000
91120 Jerusalem
Israel

V Gross
Innere Medizin II
Klinikum St. Marien Amberg
Mariahilfbergweg 7
D-92224 Amberg
Germany

OFW James
University of Newcastle
The Medical School
Centre for Liver Research
Framlington Place
Newcastle upon Tyne, NE2 4HH
United Kingdom

R Keller
Medizin Klinik II
Klinikum Aschaffenburg
Am Hasenkopf
D-63739 Aschaffenburg
Germany

A-J Kroesen
Department of Surgery
Charité – Campus Benjamin Franklin
Hindenburgdamm 30
D-12203 Berlin
Germany

U Leuschner
Internistisches Facharztzentrum
Stresemannallee 3
D-60596 Frankfurt
Germany

A Levine
E Wolfson Medical Center
Pediatric Gastroenterology and
  Nutrition
PO Box 5
58100 Holon
Israel

MP Manns
Department of Gastroenterology,
  Hepatology and Endocrinology
Medizinische Hochschule Hannover
Carl-Neuberg-Str. 1
D-30625 Hannover
Germany

AS Peña
Vrije Universiteit
Faculteit der Geneeskunde
Gastrointestinale & Immunogenetic
Van der Boechorststraat 7
1081 BT Amsterdam
The Netherlands

M Raithel
Innere Medizin I
Universität Erlangen-Nürnberg
Ulmenweg 18
D-91054 Erlangen
Germany

P Reichardt
Medizinische Klinik mit Schwerpunkt
  Hematologie und Onkologie
Campus Virchow Klinikum des
  Universitätsklinikum Charité
Augustenburger Platz 1
D-13353 Berlin
Germany

J-D Schulzke
Innere Medizin I
Universitätsklinikum Benjamin
  Franklin der Freien Universität
  Berlin
Hindenburgdamm 30
D-12203 Berlin
Germany

OØ Thomsen
Department of Gastroenterology C
Herlev Hospital
University of Copenhagen
Herlev Ringvej 75
D-2730 Herlev
Denmark

A Tromm
Innere Medizin
Evang. Krankenhaus Hattingen
Bredenscheider Str. 54
D-45525 Hattingen
Germany

Preface

The topical glucocorticoid budesonide has been well known for a long time in the medical community because of its beneficial effects in the treatment of chronic obstructive pulmonary diseases. Budesonide is characterized by a high first-pass effect and a rapid metabolism in the liver, resulting in low systemic bioavailability and, compared to conventional glucocorticoids, a reduced frequency of side-effects. For about a decade now, budesonide has been used by gastroenterologists and it has been proven especially effective in the treatment of distal ulcerative colitis and ileocolonic Crohn's disease in a number of randomized controlled clinical studies. In recent years budesonide has also been successfully used in the management of other diseases in the fields of gastroenterology, hepatology, surgery and oncology.

The aim of this workshop on budesonide was to critically discuss the current role of budesonide in gastroenterology, hepatology, surgery and oncology. The use of budesonide for the treatment of distal ulcerative colitis and ileocolonic Crohn's disease was evaluated in detail with respect to its role in an evidence-based management of IBD. A main focus was put on potential new indications for the use of budesonide, as a number of smaller clinical studies and anecdotal case reports with impressive clinical effects have been reported in patients with gastrointestinal, hepatic, oncological and surgical problems. Finally, as our clinical experience with the use of budesonide is increasing, safety issues and the side-effect profile of budesonide were addressed.

The editors would like to thank all authors for their timely contributions, which made rapid publication of the proceedings of this meeting possible. These contributions certainly reflect the current state of the art in the use of budesonide in gastroenterology, surgery, oncology and hepatology. The editors are indebted to Ursula and Dr. Dr. Herbert Falk and the Falk Foundation, Freiburg, for their generous support and the exceptional organization of the meeting. Furthermore, we wish to thank Ms. Linda Thomas and Mr. Phil Johnstone, Lancaster Publishing Services Ltd., for their help and cooperation in preparing this volume.

A. Dignass
H.J. Buhr
V. Gross
O.F.W. James

Section I
Evidence-based use of budesonide in gastroenterology and hepatology

1
Mode of action and pharmacokinetics

A. TROMM

INTRODUCTION

Glucocorticoids have been used for the first-line treatment of inflammatory bowel disease (IBD) for nearly 50 years. The efficacy of glucocorticoids to induce remission in IBD mainly depends on their various anti-inflammatory effects[1].

The synopsis of therapeutic studies on glucocorticoids over the years shows a trend towards a more rational glucocorticoid therapy. For a long period of time C_{21} alcohols (hydrocortisone, methylprednisolone, prednisolone, betamethasone) were used as 'classic' glucocorticoids. Furthermore, glucocorticoid esters (hydrocortisone phosphate, methylprednisolone hemisuccinate, prednisolone hemisuccinate, betamethasone phosphate) have been introduced as prodrugs for systemic and topical use. Since 10 years ago budesonide, beclomethasone dipropionate, fluticasone and hydrocortisone thiopivalate have been of interest for the targeted therapy of IBD[2,3]. Currently budesonide is the drug of choice for the topical treatment of IBD by oral and rectal application.

MODE OF ACTION, PHARMACODYNAMICS

After *oral* application systemically acting glucocorticoids are absorbed in the upper small bowel and pass into the cytoplasm of the target cells to develop their genomic or non-genomic functions[4–6]. Moreover, glucocorticoids given in higher doses induce unspecific effects.

The glucocorticoid receptor (GR) consists of about 770 amino acids throughout the human body and can be divided into three domains. The GR is associated with two molecules of heat-shock protein 90. Receptor binding of the GR leads to a change of the conformation and – depending on temperature – to a dissociation of GR and the heat-shock protein. The activated GR can pass into the nucleus and modulates gene transcription. It has been estimated that up to 100 genes can be regulated by glucocorticoids[7,8]. In detail, binding of GR to DNA enhances the synthesis of lipocortin-1. Lipocortin-1 inhibits phospholipase A_2 and the targets of the arachidonic cascade (prostaglandins, leucotrienes, platelet-activating factor).

Table 1 Glucocorticoids: mode of action

Glucocorticosteroid receptor binding induces lipocortin synthesis
   → lipocortin-1 ↑
   → inhibition of phospholipase A_2
   → inhibition of prostaglandins (PGE_2)
   → inhibition of leucotrienes (LTB_4)
   → inhibition of platelet-activating factor

Different reactions depend on direct protein–protein interactions or binding of the ligand to a membrane-binding receptor[9]. Binding to glucocorticoid-responsive elements also leads to diverging effects on gene transcription by inhibition and activation.

For the treatment of IBD the interactions between glucocorticoids and cells or mediators of the inflammatory cascade are most relevant[10–12]. However, the different modes of action of the glucocorticoids have not been investigated completely.

Granulocytes

After oral or intravenous application glucocorticoids lead to a 2–3-fold increase of circulating neutrophil granulocytes, whereas the number of circulating monocytes, lymphocytes and basophils decreases[13]. It has been a matter of discussion whether this effect depends on an increased release of neutrophils from the bone marrow or a decreased migration of neutrophils[14].

Lymphocytes

The decrease of peripheral lymphocytes after application of glucocorticoids expresses the distribution of lymphocytes into lymphatic organs (e.g. spleen, lymph nodes)[15]. The inhibitory effect of glucocorticoids on T lymphocytes is stronger than on B lymphocytes[16].

Monocytes, macrophages

Glucocorticoids lead to a marked decrease of monocytes and macrophages of the peripheral blood by redistribution[17]. Subsequently the macrophage-induced synthesis of prostaglandins declines[18].

Adhesion molecules, endothelial cells

The interactions of leucocytes and endothelial cells are mediated by adhesion molecules (ICAM-1, ELAM-1 or VCAM-1). Glucocorticoids inhibit the enhanced expression of ICAM-1 by macrophages and the accumulation of leucocytes at the site of inflammation, and reduce the histamine-mediated acceleration of permeability[19,20].

Table 2 Effect of glucocorticoids on peripheral blood cells

Increase (2–3-fold) of neutrophils

Decrease of monocytes
Decrease of lymphocytes
Decrease of eosinophils
Decrease of basophils

Table 3 Effect of glucocorticoids on cytokines

Inhibition of:

   Interleukin-1
   Interleukin-2
   Interleukin-6
   Interleukin-8
   TNF-alpha

Cytokines

Glucocorticoids also inhibit numerous proinflammatory cytokines, e.g. interleukin-1[21,22] and tumour necrosis factor alpha[23]. With respect to a post-transcriptional inhibition of m-RNA[24], glucocorticoids regulate the expression of interleukin-2[25], interleukin-6[26] and interleukin-8[27]. In IBD an inhibition of the release of interleukin-1 from colonic mucosa after incubation with prednisolone has been described[28]. Braegger et al.[29] described a decrease of tumour necrosis factor alpha in faeces during glucocorticoid therapy. In addition, the inhibition of prostaglandin E_2 and leukotriene B_4 by prednisolone – via lipocortin – has been shown *in vivo*[30,31].

Glucocorticoid receptor (GR) in IBD

GR levels in peripheral blood mononuclear cells (PBMC) are significantly decreased in GC-treated patients vs controls ($p = 0.002$) and patients not treated with GC ($p = 0.007$). Mucosal GR levels were found to be decreased independently of treatment[32]. Expression of the GR (PBMC) was suppressed to normal levels under steroid treatment, but K_d remained elevated[33]. IBD patients without steroids showed a significant increase both in the expression of GR per cell and in the apparent dissociation constant[33]. The amounts of GRα-mRNA and GRβ-mRNA (PBMC) in Crohn's disease patients were lower ($p < 0.05$) than those of the healthy subjects. In addition, an inverse correlation between the duration of the disease and GRα-mRNA has been described[34].

Effects on impaired ion transport systems

The positive influence of GC on various impaired ion transport systems has been demonstrated in several animal studies (for overview see ref. 35).

In detail, changes in sodium–amino acid transport[36], Cl^-/HCO_3^- transport[37], uptake of sodium + glucose[38], Na^+/K^+ exchange[39] and electrolyte transport[40,41] have been shown. Ecker and co-workers[35] showed that the absorptive capacity of the intestinal mucosa for water may be improved by budesonide. This effect occurs independently of the anti-inflammatory effect.

In general, glucocorticoids can inhibit inflammatory reactions by interaction with numerous cells and different mediators within the inflammatory cascade of ulcerative colitis and Crohn's disease.

BUDESONIDE

Budesonide is a non-halogenated, lipophilic steroid which shows a relatively high receptor-binding affinity (RBA = 845) as compared to dexamethasone (RBA = 100)[42]. The RBA of budesonide is 20-fold higher than that of methylprednisolone (RBA = 42). The active form is a C_{21} alcohol. The distribution (2.8–4.3 L/kg) is relatively high as compared to conventional glucocorticoids, and argues for a high tissue affinity[43,44]. About 88% of budesonide was bound to albumin; 90% of budesonide was inactivated during the first-pass effect in the liver by cytochrome P450[45,46]. The resulting metabolites, 6β-OH-budesonide and 16α-OH-predniso-lone, show less than 1% of the intrinsic activity of budesonide, and do not induce any systemic activity[47,48]. The high plasma-clearance of 1.2 L/min underlines the rapid metabolism.

Table 4 Characteristics of budesonide

Non-halogenated glucocorticoid
Highly lipophilic
C_{16}–C_{17}-acetonide
C_{21} alcohol
High receptor-binding affinity
High first-pass effect
High plasma clearance
Low bioavailability

The low bioavailability of budesonide (11%) depends mainly on the high first-pass effect in the liver. Together with the enhanced mucosal dwell time as compared to prednisolone, budesonide comprises advantages for the topical therapy of IBD with GC.

Experimental data from Miller-Larsson et al.[49] revealed evidence that budesonide has an enhanced residence time in colonic mucosa as compared to prednisolone; 20 min and 4 h after perfusion of the rat colon significantly higher concentrations of budesonide (15-fold or 50-fold) were detected as compared to prednisolone. The concentrations were found to be 10-fold higher in the mucosa than in the submucosa.

For practical use a galenic preparation leading to a targeted delivery of budesonide at the site of inflammation is required. Coating with eudragit –

similiar to 5-aminosalicylic acid (5-ASA) – formulations has been introduced for budesonide to realize a pH-modified release[8].

The pH-modified-release formulation (Budenofalk[®]) consists of a hard gelatine capsule which contains about 400 pellets with a diameter of approximately 1 mm. Each pellet consists of a sugar matrix with an outer budesonide drug layer. Because of being small, the pellets leave the stomach continuously. In contrast, tablets – with a larger diameter – are delivered to the duodenum only during phase III of the migrating motor complex. The delivery of budesonide has been realized by a pH-dependent delivery system using eudragit coating which has been established for 5-ASA preparations.

PHARMACOKINETICS

Studies from our group (HW Möllmann, AC Möllmann, M Wagner, G Hochhaus, H Derendorf, and A Tromm) investigated the pharmacokinetics and pharmacodynamics of budesonide in different drug formulations in single and multiple dosages once or three times a day at 8-h intervals[2].

The concentration–time profiles are shown in Figures 1 and 2. Application of eudragit-coated Budenofalk[®] capsules at different doses (3×1 mg, 3×2 mg, 3×3 mg) leads to marked delay of resorption after 2–4 h as compared to tablets (Figure 1). Thus, the resorption of budesonide occurs with a significant time lag. In contrast, application of plain tablets leads to an immediate release without any time lag (Figure 2).

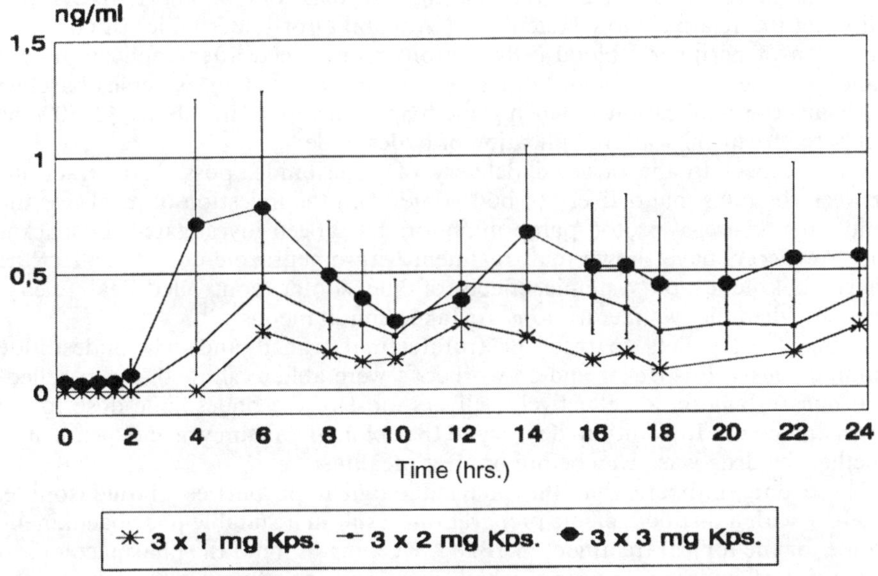

Figure 1 Concentration–time profiles (HPLC–RIA) after application of budesonide pH-modified release capsules 1, 2 and 3 mg in healthy volunteers ($n = 12$)

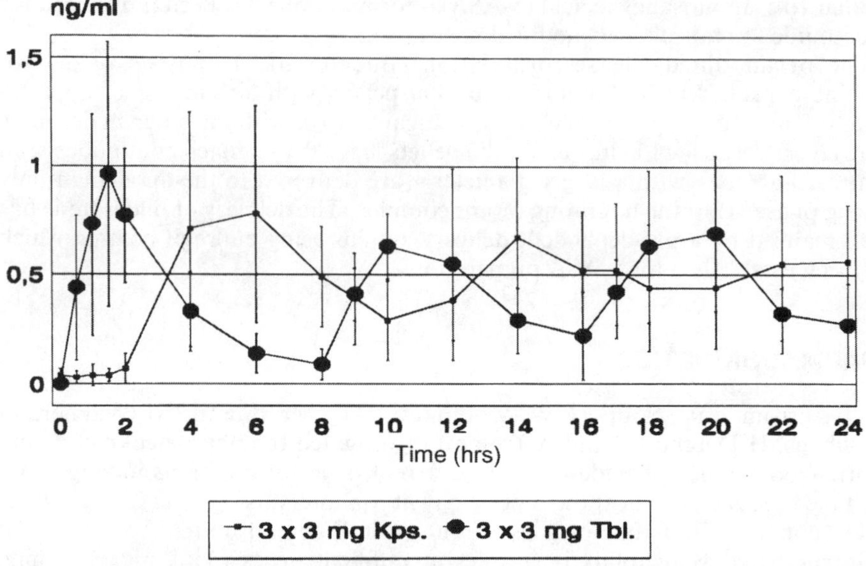

Figure 2 Concentration–time profiles (HPLC–RIA) after application of budesonide pH-modified release capsules 3 mg vs tablets 3 mg in healthy volunteers ($n = 12$)

A slight increase of neutrophils and a slight decrease of lymphocytes is evident, reflecting the relatively low systemic bioavailability of budesonide. In contrast, alteration of peripheral blood cells is more pronounced after application of a standard dose of methylprednisolone. The quantitative changes versus baseline following the application of 40 mg methylprednisolone are about 40–50% as compared to 20–30% after application of budesonide[50].

With respect to the targeted delivery of budesonide, possible interactions between the intestinal delivery of budesonide and the ingestion of meals, or the simultaneous use of proton-pump inhibitors have been investigated. Edsbäcker and co-workers have shown that treatment with omeprazole does not affect the pharmacokinetics or systemic effects of budesonide controlled-ileal release capsules when the two medications are taken simultaneously[51].

Using ^{111}In pellets to trace gastrointestinal transit and $^2H_8$ budesonide simultaneously, Edsbäcker and co-workers[52] were able to show that controlled-ileal release budesonide effectively delivers most of the budesonide dose to the ileum and colon. In addition, delivery to the colon and ileum was independent of whether the drug was given before or after breakfast[52].

These data indicate that the pharmacological properties of budesonide, together with a distinct galenic preparation, result in a suitable pharmacokinetic profile for the topical treatment of IBD[53]. Keeping in mind the pharmacological properties of budesonide with the high local and low systemic availability, the ideal subgroups of patients for budesonide treatment of IBD (e.g. location, activity) have to be identified. Thus, budesonide leads to an improvement of IBD therapy.

References

1. Meyers S. Oral and parenteral corticoids. In: Peppercorn MA, editor. Therapy of Inflammatory Bowel Disease. New York: Marcel Dekker, 1990:3–33.
2. Möllmann HW, Barth J, Hochhaus G, Mölmann AC, Derendorf H, Tromm A. Principles of topical versus systemic corticoid treatment in inflammatory bowel disease. In: Möllmann HW, May B, editors. Glucocorticoid Therapy in Chronic Inflammatory Bowel Disease. Dordrecht: Kluwer, 1996:1–14.
3. Tromm A, Möllmann HW, May B. Glucocorticoid therapy practice in chronic inflammatory bowel disease. Results of a survey of German therapeutic centres. In: Möllmann HW, May B, editors. Glucocorticoid Therapy in Chronic Inflammatory Bowel Disease. Dordrecht: Kluwer, 1996:1–14.
4. Milsap RL, George DE, Szefler SJ, Murray KA, Lebenthal E, Jusko WJ. Effect of inflammatory bowel disease on absorption and disposition of prednisolone. Dig Dis Sci. 1983;28:161–8.
5. Rugstad HE. Antiinflammatory and immunoregulatory effects of glucocorticoids: mode of action. Scand J Rheumatol. 1988;76:257–64.
6. Tanner AR, Halliday JW, Powell LW. Serum prednisolone levels in Crohn's disease and celiac disease following oral prednisolone administration. Digestion. 1981;21:310–15.
7. Brattsand R. Steroid development: a case of enhanced selectivity for the bowel wall. In: Jewell DP, Rutgeerts P, editors. Reviewing Steroids in the Treatment of IBD. Res Clin Forums. 1993;15:17–31.
8. Hochhaus G, Derendorf H, Möllmann HW, Barth J, Hochhaus R. Pharmacodynamic aspects of glucocoticoid action. In: May B, Möllmann HW, editors. Glucocorticoid Therapy in Chronic Inflammatory Bowel Disease. Dordrecht: Kluwer, 1996:61–79.
9. Müller M, Renkawitz R. The glucocorticoid receptor. Biochem Biophys Acta. 1991;1088:171–82.
10. Andus T, Targan SR. Glucocorticoids. In: Targan SR, Shanahan F, editors. Inflammatory Bowel Disease. From Bench to Bedside. Baltimore: Williams & Wilkins, 1994:487–502.
11. Kuritzkes RA, Shanahan F. Corticosteroid therapy. In: Gitnick G, editor. Inflammatory Bowel Disease. Diagnosis and Treatment. Tokyo: Igaku-Shoin, 1991:299–321.
12. Parente L, Mugridge KG. Glucocorticoids and gastrointestinal inflammation. In: Wallace JL, editor. Immunopharmacology of the Gastrointestinal System. London: Academic Press, 1993:169–84.
13. Mishler JM, Benedict CR. Dexamethasone-induced neutrophilia. Negative correlation with increased plasma adrenaline concentrations. Experientia. 1978;34:259–60.
14. Cupps TR, Fauci AS. Corticosteroid-mediated immunoregulation in man. Immunol Rev. 1982;65:133–55.
15. Bloemena E, Weinreich S, Schellekens PT. The influence of prednisolone on the recirculation of peripheral blood lymphocytes in $vivo$. Clin Exp Immunol. 1990;80:460–6.
16. Verbrüggen G, Herman L, Ackerman C, Mielants H, Veys EM. The effect of low doses of prednisolone on T-cell subsets in rheumatoid arthritis. Int J Immunopharmacol. 1987;9:1–67.
17. Thompson J, van Furth R. The effect of glucocorticosteroids on the kinetics of mononuclear phagocytes. J Exp Med. 1970;131:429–42.
18. Werb Z. Biochemical actions of glucocorticoids on macrophages in culture. Specific inhibition of elastase, collagenase, and plasminogen activator secretion and effects on other metabolic functions. J Exp Med. 1978;147:1695–712.
19. Watanabe M, Yagi M, Omata M. Stimulation of neutrophil adherence to vascular endothelial cells by histamine and thrombin and its inhibition by PAF antagonists and dexamethasone. Br J Pharmacol. 1991;102:239–45.
20. Wiiliams TJ, Yarwood H. Effect of glucocorticoids on microvascular permeability. Am Rev Respir Dis. 1990;141:S39–43.
21. Lee SW, Tsou A-P, Chad H, Thomas J, Petrie K, Eugui EM, Allison AC. Glucocorticoids selectively inhibit the transcription of the interleukin 1β gene and decrease the stability of interleukin 1β mRNA. Proc Natl Acad Sci USA. 1988;85:1204–8.
22. Lew W, Oppenheim JJ, Matsushima K. Analysis of the suppression of IL-1α and IL-1β production in human peripheral blood mononuclear adherent cells by a glucocorticoid hormone. J Immunol. 1988;140:1895–902.

23. Beutler B, Cerami A. Cachectin and tumor necrosis factor as two sides of the same biological coin. Nature. 1986;320:584–8.
24. Tobler A, Meier R, Seitz M, Dewald B, Bagglionini M, Fey FF. Gluococorticoids down-regulate gene expression of GM-CSF, NAP-1/Il-8 and Il-6, but not M-CSF in human fibroblasts. Blood. 1992;79:45–51.
25. Smith KA. T-cell growth factor. Immunol Rev. 1980;51:337–57.
26. Helfgott DC, May LT, Sthoeger Z, Tamm I, Segal PB. Bacterial lipopolysaccharide (endotoxin) enhances expression and secretion of β_2 interferon by human fibroblasts. J Exp Med. 1987;166:1300–9.
27. Mukaida N, Shiroo M, Matsushima K. Genomic structure of the human monocyte-derived neutrophil chemotactic factor IL-8. J Immunol. 1989;143:1366–71.
28. Rachmilewitz D, Eliakim R, Simon P, Ligumsky M, Karmeli F. Cytokines and platelet-activating factor in human inflamed colonic mucosa. Agents Actions Suppl. 1992;36:C32–6.
29. Braegger CP, Nichols S, Murch SH, Stephens S, McDonald TT. Tumor necrosis factor alpha in stool as a marker of intestinal inflammation. Lancet. 1992;338:89–91.
30. Lauritsen K, Laursen LS, Bukhave K, Rask-Madsen J. Effects of topical 5-aminosalicylic acid and prednisolone on prostaglandin E_2 and leukotriene B_4 levels determined by equilibrium *in vivo* dialysis of rectum in relapsing ulcerative colitis. Gastroenterology. 1986;91:837–44.
31. Lauritsen K, Laursen LS, Bukhave K, Rask-Madsen J. *In vivo* effects of orally administered prednisolone on prostaglandin and leukotriene production in ulcerative colitis. Gut. 1987;28: 1095–9.
32. Rogler G, Meinel A, Lingauer A et al. Glucocorticoid receptors are down-regulated in inflamed colonic mucosa but not in peripheral blood mononuclear cells from patients with inflammatory bowel disease. Eur J Clin Invest. 1999;29:330–6.
33. Schottelius A, Wedel S, Weltrich R et al. Higher expression of glucocorticoid receptor in peripheral mononuclear cells in inflammatory bowel disease. Am J Gastroenterol. 2000;95: 1994–9.
34. Hori T, Watanabe K, Miyaoki M, Moriyasu F, Onda K, Hirano T, Oka K. Glucocorticoid receptors and Crohn's disease. Expression of mRNA for glucocorticoid receptors in peripheral blood mononuclear cells of patients with Crohn's disease. J Gastroenterol Hepatol. 2002;17:1070–7.
35. Ecker K-W, Stallmach A, Seitz G, Greinwald R, Achenbach U. Oral budesonide significantly improves water absorption in patients with ileostomy for Crohn's disease. Scand J Gastro-enterol. 2003;38:288–93.
36. Hua A, Weisel S, Sundaram U. Glucocorticoid mediated reversal of Na^+ amino acid co-transport inhibition during chronic ileitis. Gastroenterology. 1999;116:A935 (abstract).
37. Coon S, Sundaram U. Mechanism of glucocorticoid mediated reversal of Na:Cl absorption inhibition during chronic ileitis. Gastroenterology. 1999;116:A935 (abstract).
38. Thiesen A, Tappenden KA, McBurney MI, Clandinin MT, Keelan M, Wild G. The effect of locally and systemically active steroids on the transport of sugars following intestinal resection in rats is influenced by dietary lipids. Gastroenterology. 1997;112:A910 (abstract).
39. Bastl CP, Schulman G, Cragoe EJ. Low-dose glucocorticoids stimulate electroneutral NaCl absorption in rat colon. Am J Physiol. 1989;257:1027–38.
40. Sandle GI. Segmental variability of glucocorticoid induced electrolyte transport in rat colon. Gut. 1991;32:936–40.
41. Turnamian SG, Binder HJ. Regulation of active sodium and potassium transport in the distal colon of the rat. J Clin Invest. 1989;84:1924–9.
42. Möllmann HW, Hochhaus G, Tromm A et al. Topical use of steroids in gastroenterology. In: Schölmerich J, Kruis W, Goebell H, Hohenberger W, Gross V, editors. Inflammatory Bowel Diseases – Pathophysiology as Basis of Treatment. Dordrecht: Kluwer, 1993:343–9.
43. Edsbäcker S, Johansson S-A. Correlation between kinetic properties and clinical safety of budesonide enema. Abstracts of the World Congress of Gastroenterology, Sydney, 1990; Medicine Group (UK), Abingdon: PD 561 (abstract).
44. Ryrfeldt A, Andersson P, Edsbäcker S, Tönnesson M, Davies D, Paulwels R. Pharmacoki-netics and metabolism of budesonide, a selective glucocorticoid. Eur J Resp Dis. 1982;63 (Suppl. 122):86–95.
45. Edsbäcker S, Anderson P, Lindberg C, Paulson J, Ryrfeldt A, Thalen A. Metabolic acetal splitting of budesonide – a novel inactivation pathway for topical glucocorticoids. Drug Metab Dispos. 1987;15:651–5.

46. Jönsson G, Astrom A, Andersson P. Budesonide is metabolized by cytochrome P450 (CYPA3A) enzymes in human liver. Drug Metab Dispos. 1995;23:137–42.
47. Edsbäcker S. Studies on the metabolic fate and human pharmacokinetics of budesonide. Thesis, Lund University, Sweden, 1986.
48. Edsbäcker S, Jönsson S, Lindberg C, Ryrfeldt A, Thalen, A. Metabolic pathways of the topical glucocorticoid budesonide in man. Drug Metab Dispos. 1983;11:590–6.
49. Miller-Larsson A, Gustafsson B, Persson CGA, Brattsand R. Gut mucosal uptake and retention characteristics contribute the high intestinal selectivity of budesonide compared with prednisolone in the rat. Aliment Pharmacol Ther. 2001;15:2019–25.
50. Barth J, Damoiseaux M, Möllmann H, Brandis K-H, Hochhaus G, Derendorf H. Pharmacokinetics and pharmacodynamics of prednisolone after intravenous and oral administration. Int J Clin Pharmacol Ther. 1992;30:317–24.
51. Edsbäcker S, Larsson P, Bergstrand M. Pharmacokinetics of budesonide controlled-release capsules when taken with omeprazole. Aliment Pharmacol Ther. 12003;7:403–8.
52. Edsbäcker S, Larsson P, Wolmer P. Gut delivery of budesonide, a locally active corticosteroid, from plain and controlled-release capsules. Eur J Gastroenterol Hepatol. 2002;14:1357–62.
53. Baker DE. Budesonide modified-release capsules. Rev Gastroenterol Disord. 2001;1:147–55.

2
Safety profile and potential side-effects of budesonide

O. Ø THOMSEN

INTRODUCTION

Budesonide is a glucocorticosteroid with a weak mineralocorticosteroid activity. It has a favourable ratio between anti-inflammatory activity and systemic glucocorticosteroid effect over a wide dose range. This is explained by a high local glucocorticosteroid activity and an extensive first-pass hepatic degradation to metabolites with very low glucococorticosteroid activity. Due to these circumstances the well-known glucocorticosteroid adverse effects[1] are less frequent with budesonide treatment than with the conventional corticosteroids. Budesonide has been used for several years in the treatment of chronic inflammatory bowel diseases, especially with oral treatment of active Crohn's disease and enema treatment of active distal ulcerative colitis.

This chapter highlights the safety results of studies with short-term and long-term treatment with budesonide in patients with Crohn's disease and ulcerative colitis, and focuses on the results of double-blind, randomized, clinical controlled trials.

ADVERSE EVENTS IN SHORT-TERM STUDIES

Budesonide versus placebo for treatment of active Crohn's disease

Two randomized controlled 8-week studies have been performed comparing budesonide therapy with placebo in patients with active Crohn's disease[2,3]. Both studies showed no statistically significant difference in the total number of adverse events and the total number of glucocorticosteroid-associated adverse events between the budesonide and the placebo treatment groups. Furthermore, a meta-analysis of these two studies gave the same results[4,5], and the odds ratio of glucocorticosteroid-associated side-effects was 0.98[5].

Budesonide versus conventional corticosteroids for treatment of active Crohn's disease

Five randomized, double-blind clinical controlled studies with treatment duration of 8–12 weeks comparing budesonide with conventional corticosteroid therapy in active Crohn's disease have been published[6–10]. Meta-analyses of all these studies showed statistically significantly fewer glucocorticosteroid-associated adverse events in the budesonide group compared with conventional corticosteroids (i.e. prednisolone or 6-methylprednisolone)[4,5]. The odds ratio of glucocorticosteroid-related side-effects was 0.39 in favour of budesonide in the meta-analysis of Otley et al.[5] and 0.65 in a meta-analysis of Kane et al.[4]. The latter meta-analysis, however, included a trial with open treatment[11].

ADVERSE EVENTS IN LONG-TERM STUDIES

Budesonide versus placebo for maintenance of remission in Crohn's disease

Six randomized controlled trials, all with budesonide versus placebo treatment for 1 year, have been published. Four of the trials were in patients with medically induced remission[12–15] and two studies on the prevention of postsurgical recurrence[16–17]. The total number of adverse events, or the proportion of patients reporting such events, was not significantly different in the budesonide and placebo groups. The total number of glucocorticosteroid-associated side-effects was higher (n.s.) in some of the studies[12,13,15], but not in others[16]. Moon face and acne[15] or bruising[12] were slightly more frequent in some of the studies, but not in others. The frequency of some events diminished in parallel in both treatment groups during the study duration, and this may be explained by the pre-study medication. The good tolerability of long-term use of budesonide from these studies is supported by the data from compassionate use in over 4000 patients, in some for more than 5 years, and the post-marketing surveillance[18].

Budesonide or placebo for maintenance of remission in quiescent Crohn's disease

Two randomized controlled studies in patients with steroid-dependent disease have been published; one study with treatment duration of 22 weeks[19] and another lasting 1 year[20]. In these studies no significant differences in adverse events or glucocorticosteroid-associated adverse events were found between the budesonide (6 mg daily) and the control groups (placebo[19] or mesalamine[20]).

BUDESONIDE VERSUS MESALAMINE THERAPY FOR ACTIVE OR QUIESCENT CROHN'S DISEASE

Two randomized trials have been published comparing treatment with budesonide and mesalamine[20,21] for Crohn's disease. In the study by Thomsen et al.[21]

patients with active disease (CDAI 200–400) were treated with budesonide 9 mg daily or mesalamine 4 g daily for 16 weeks. In the study by Mantzaris et al.[20] patients with quiescent steroid-dependent disease (CDAI < 150) were treated for up to 1 year with either budesonide 6 mg daily or mesalamine 3 g daily. In both studies no significant difference in the total number of adverse events was found[20,21]. However, the number of severe adverse events was more frequent with mesalamine treatment than with budesonide[21].

From the randomized controlled trials it can be concluded that no significant difference in the frequency of glucocorticosteroid-associated adverse events has been observed for patients treated with budesonide compared with placebo or mesalamine. Furthermore, fewer glucocorticosteroid adverse events were found in patients treated with budesonide compared to conventional corticosteroid therapy. Corticosteroid-dependent patients treated with budesonide were more likely to maintain remission than patients treated with placebo or mesalamine. Therefore, long-term treatment with budesonide may be valuable for long-term management of patients with glucocorticosteroid-dependent Crohn's disease. Long-term effects of budesonide treatment, and also combination therapy with immunosuppressors, need to be elucidated.

EFFECTS OF BUDESONIDE ON QUALITY OF LIFE

Several randomized controlled studies have shown significant improvement of budesonide treatment on health-related quality of life indices in patients with Crohn's disease[9,19,20,22,23]. Thus, the Inflammatory Bowel Disease Questionnaire (IBDQ) score and the Psychological General Well-Being (PGWB) index, together with a number of subcomponents to these indices, all improved significantly during budesonide treatment compared to placebo[22] and treatment with mesalamine 3 or 4 g daily[20,21,23].

EFFECT OF BUDESONIDE ON ADRENAL GLAND FUNCTION

The plasma cortisol level only partly reflects adrenal gland function. Adrenal gland suppression can be more precisely determined by testing its response to adrenocorticotropic hormone (ACTH). This method gives a measure of the functional reserve of the adrenal gland for glucocorticosteroid secretion.

Ulcerative colitis

In the treatment of active ulcerative colitis budesonide enema 2 mg daily for up to 8 weeks has been shown not to influence plasma cortisol levels[24]. This is in contrast to the results of treatment with other steroid enemas such as hydrocortisone[25], methylprednisolone[26] and prednisolone[24,27–29]. The ACTH-stimulated cortisol response may be reduced in up to 10% of such patients treated with budesonide enema for 6–8 weeks[30,31]; this, however, is less frequent compared to enema treatment with hydrocortisone[29], or prednisolone[30] for only a few weeks.

Crohn's disease

In the 8–10-week trials in patients with active Crohn's disease the plasma cortisol level showed a dose-dependent decrease during treatment with oral budesonide 3, 6, 9, or 15 mg daily[32]. Thus, the lowering effect on plasma cortisol level of budesonide 15 mg daily was not significantly different from that of prednisolone 40 mg daily. A much smaller effect on plasma cortisol was found with budesonide 9 mg daily. With this budesonide dose approximately one-third of the patients had abnormal plasma cortisol level[6,21] and 10%[21] and 58%[8] of the patients had impaired adrenal gland function as estimated by ACTH tests. The corresponding figure from the ACTH test for prednisolone treatment was 84%[8]. In the 1-year studies with budesonide 3 mg or 6 mg daily many patients normalized their pre-study abnormal plasma cortisol level and only a few patients had subnormal plasma cortisol values and subnormal ACTH tests after treatment for 1 year[13,16].

Thus, budesonide treatment may affect adrenal gland function, but mostly to a small extent. The majority of patients have normal plasma cortisol level and respond normally to ACTH stimulation. Pre-study abnormal adrenal gland function (due to treatment with conventional glucocorticosteroids) may even be normalized during long-term therapy with budesonide 3 or 6 mg daily.

OF SPECIAL INTEREST

Bone metabolism

More data on the effect of long-term treatment with budesonide on bone metabolism are required. The existing data, however, suggest that the risk of e.g. osteoporosis is lower after budesonide treatment than after prednisolone. In the study of D'Haens et al.[11] on bone metabolism in patients with Crohn's disease treated with budesonide or methylprednisolone for 10 weeks the markers of bone degradation and synthesis were not impaired in the budesonide group. Serum osteocalcin values were unchanged after 8 weeks of budesonide 9 mg daily in patients with active Crohn's disease[9]. In patients with quiescent Crohn's disease with prospective annual measurements of bone mineral density for 2 years budesonide did not show any advantage over low-dose prednisone for preservation of bone mineral density[33]. However, the loss of bone mineral density was significantly less with budesonide flexible dosing up to 9 mg daily compared to prednisolone with treatment for up to 2 years in patients with steroid-naive Crohn's disease[34]. Furthermore, in primary biliary cirrhosis bone mineral density did not change significantly after treatment with budesonide 9 mg daily for 2 years in comparison with a control group and the pre-treatment status[35].

Psychiatric events

Pooled data from five short-term and five long-term randomized studies in patients with Crohn's disease have been integrated for safety analysis[36]. The short-term studies including 772 patients with active Crohn's disease showed a significantly reduced frequency of any preferred symptom from body system psychiatric disorders in the budesonide group compared to prednisolone. From the pooled data of long-term studies on 417 patients with Crohn's disease in remission 14% and 16% of the patients had any psychiatric symptom in the placebo and the budesonide group, respectively (n.s.). Furthermore, in the 8-week and the 1-year studies from this safety analysis the frequency of insomnia, mood swings and depression was similar in patients treated with budesonide and placebo.

Children

Published data on oral budesonide therapy in children are limited. The systemic exposure to budesonide in children with active Crohn's disease has been investigated in a pharmacokinetic study and compared to findings in adults[37]. The systemic exposure (AUC-24 h), systemic availability ($9 \pm 5\%$) and cortisol suppression were of the same order of magnitude in children and adults.

One randomized double-blind controlled study of budesonide 9 mg daily versus prednisolone 40 mg daily in 48 children aged 6–16 years with active Crohn's disease has been performed[10]. In this 12-week study budesonide was well tolerated at doses normally given to adults and with significantly fewer gluco-corticosteroid-associated adverse events than seen with prednisolone treatment (23% versus 60%). At 8 weeks 63% of the patients in the budesonide group had abnormal adrenal gland function tests compared with 89% in the prednisolone group.

Pregnancy

The toxicology profile of budesonide has been thoroughly tested in several species of animals over a wide range of doses[18]. The results have shown similar effects to glucocorticosteroids on toxicological effects, fertility and reproduction. Standard tests have failed to reveal any mutagenic properties associated with budesonide. Clinical experience with oral budesonide therapy in pregnancy is limited. However, the incidence of malformations is unchanged in budesonide-treated asthmatic women[18].

Breast-feeding women

The clinical experience with oral budesonide therapy is limited in breast-feeding women, but it appears to be well tolerated. Glucocorticosteroids are excreted in breast milk. The calculated dose passed on to the child is only 0.05–0.25% of the dose to the mother[18].

Impaired liver function

Impaired hepatic function may increase the systemic bioavailability of budeso-nide due to reduced hepatic biotransformation. Clinical experience of budeso-nide in liver diseases is limited, but oral treatment with budesonide 9 mg daily for up to 2 years showed excellent tolerability in the study of Leucshner et al.[35] in 40 patients with primary biliary cirrhosis. Conversion to budesonide treatment with

9 mg daily in steroid-dependent autoimmune hepatitis has been unsuccessful due to withdrawal symptoms and treatment failure[38].

Miscellaneous

Budesonide treatment in chronic inflammatory bowel diseases in short-term and long-term studies did not show any significant change in mean pulse rate, blood pressure, or biochemical and haematological variables. Standard tests have failed to reveal any mutagenic properties associated with budesonide[18].

CONCLUSION

The incidence of adverse events with budesonide treatment in patients with chronic inflammatory bowel disease is similar to that seen with placebo and mesalamine. Moreover, the intensity of such adverse events with budesonide treatment is mostly mild or moderate, and the profile of the adverse events during budesonide therapy is representative for glucocorticosteroids. Moreover, no new adverse events with budesonide therapy compared to already well-known side-effects from the use of systemic-acting glucocorticosteroids have been reported during the use of budesonide for two decades in the treatment of chronic inflammatory bowel disease, and for a longer duration in patients with pulmonary disease. In conclusion, budesonide is well tolerated and safe for treatment of well-documented indications.

References

1. Rutgeerts PJ. Review article: The limitations of corticosteroid therapy in Crohn's disease. Aliment Pharmacol Ther. 2001;15:1515–25.
2. Greenberg GR, Feagan BR, Martin F et al. Oral budesonide for active Crohn's disease. N Engl J Med. 1994;331:836–41.
3. Tremaine WJ, Hanauer SB, Katz S et al. Budesonide CIR capsules (once or twice daily divided-dose) in active Crohn's disease: a randomised placebo-controlled study in the United States. Am J Gastroenterol. 2002;97:1748–54.
4. Kane SV, Schoenfeld P, Sandborn WJ, Tremaine W, Hofer T, Feagan BG. Systemic review: the effectiveness of budesonide therapy for Crohn's disease. Aliment Pharmacol Ther. 2002;16:1509–17.
5. Otley A, Thomson AB, Modigliani R, Thomsen OO, Steinhart H. Budesonide for induction of remission in Crohn's disease: meta-analysis of randomised controlled trials. Gastroenterology. 2003;124:A378.
6. Rutgeerts P, Löfberg R, Malchow H et al. A comparison of budesonide with prednisolone for active Crohn's disease. N Engl J Med. 1994;331:842–5.
7. Gross V, Andus T, Caesar I et al. Oral pH-modified release budesonide versus 6-methylprednisolone in active Crohn's disease. German/Austrian Budesonide Study Group. Eur J Gastroenterol Hepatol. 1996;8:905–9.
8. Camieri M, Ferguson A, Doe W, Persson T, Nilsson L-G, and the Global Budesonide Study Group. Oral budesonide is as effective as oral prednisolone in active Crohn's disease. Gut. 1997;41:209–14.
9. Bar-Meir S, Chowers Y, Lavy A et al. Budesonide versus prednisolone in the treatment of active Crohn's disease. Gastroenterology. 1998;15:835–40.
10. Escher JC, Lindquist BL, Hildebrand H et al. Budesonide capsules versus prednisolone in children with active Crohn's disease: results of a European multicenter trial. Gut. 2002;51(Suppl. III):A321.

11. D'Haens G, Verstraete A, Cheyns K, Aerden I, Bouillon R, Rutgeerts P. Bone turnover during short-term therapy with methylprednisolone or budesonide in Crohn's disease. Aliment Pharmacol Ther. 1998;12:419–24.

12. Greenberg GR, Feagan BG, Martin F et al. Oral budesonide as maintenance treatment for Crohn's disease: a placebo-controlled, dose-ranging study. Gastroenterology. 1996;110:45–51.

13. Löfberg R, Rutgeerts P, Malchow H et al. Budesonide prolongs time to relapse in ileal and ileocaecal Crohn's disease. A placebo controlled one-year study. Gut. 1996;39:82–6.

14. Gross V, Andus T, Ecker KW et al. Low dose oral pH modified release budesonide for maintenance of steroid induced remission in Crohn's disease. Gut. 1998;42:493–6.

15. Ferguson A, Campieri M, Doe W, Persson T, Nygård G, and the Global Budesonide Study Group. Oral budesonide as maintenance therapy in Crohn's disease – results of a 12-month study. Aliment Pharmacol Ther. 1998;12:175–83.

16. Hellers G, Cortot A, Jewell D et al. Oral budesonide for prevention of postsurgical recurrence in Crohn's disease. Gastroenterology. 1999;116:294–300.

17. Ewe K, Bottger T, Buhr HJ, Ecker KW, Otto HF. Low-dose budesonide treatment for prevention of postoperative recurrence of Crohn's disease: a multicentre randomized placebo-controlled trial. Eur J Gastroenterol Hepatol. 1999;11:277–82.

18. Anonymous. Safety and tolerability profile of Entocort capsules. In: Entocort Product Monograph, 3rd edn. Lund: AstraZeneca, 2001.

19. Cortot A, Colombel JF, Rutgeerts P et al. Switch from systemic steroids to budesonide in steroid dependent patients with inactive Crohn's disease. Gut. 2001;48:186–90.

20. Mantzaris GJ, Petraki K, Sfakianakis M et al. Budesonide versus mesalamine for maintaining remission in patients refusing other immunomodulators for steroid-dependent Crohn's disease. Clin Gastroenterol Hepatol. 2003;1:122–8.

21. Thomsen OØ, Cortot A, Jewell D et al. A comparison of budesonide and mesalamine for active Crohn's disease. N Engl J Med. 1998;339:370–4.

22. Irvine EJ, Greenberg GR, Feagan BG et al. Quality of life rapidly improves with budesonide therapy for active Crohn's disease. Canadian Inflammatory Bowel Disease Study Group. Inflamm Bowel Dis. 2000;6:181–7.

23. Thomsen OØ, Cortot A, Jewell D et al. Budesonide and mesalazine in active Crohn's disease: a comparison of the effects on quality of life. Am J Gastroenterol. 2002;97:649–53.

24. Löfberg R, Thomsen OØ, Langholz E et al. Budesonide versus prednisolone retention enemas in active distal ulcerative colitis. Aliment Pharmacol Ther. 1994;8:623–9.

25. Tarpila S, Turunen U, Seppälä K et al. Budesonide enema in active haemorrhagic proctitis – a controlled trial against hydrocortisone foam enema. Aliment Pharmacol Ther. 1994;8:591–5.

26. Porro GB, Prantera C, Campieri M et al. Comparative trial of methylprednisolone and budesonide enemas in active distal ulcerative colitis. Eur J Gastroenterol Hepatol. 1994;6:125–30.

27. Danielsson Å, Hellers G, Lyrenäs E, Löfberg R, Nilsson Å, Olsson O. A controlled randomized trial of budesonide versus prednisolone retention enemas in active distal ulcerative colitis. Scand J Gastroenterol. 1987;22:987–92.

28. Danish Budesonide Study Group. Budesonide enema in distal ulcerative colitis: a randomised dose-response trial with prednisolone enema as positive control. Scand J Gastroenterol. 1991;26:1225–30.

29. Bayless T. Sninsky C and the US Budesonide Enema Study Group. Budesonide enema is an effective alternative to hydrocortisone enema in active distal ulcerative colitis. Gastroenterology. 1995;108(Suppl.):A778.

30. Thomsen OØ, Andersen T, Langholz E et al. Lack of adrenal gland suppression with budesonide enema in active distal ulcerative colitis: a prednisolone-controlled 8-week study. Eur J Gastroenterol Hepatol. 1994;6:507–11.

31. Hanauer SB, Robinson M, Pruitt R et al. Budesonide enema for the treatment of active, distal ulcerative colitis or proctitis: a dose-ranging study: US budesonide enema study group. Gastroenterology. 1998;115:525–32.

32. Thomsen OØ. Safety overview of budesonide in inflammatory bowel diseases. In: Crohn's disease – Pathogenesis and Medical Therapy. Res Clin Forums. 1996;18:91–100.

33. Cino M, Greenberg GR. Bone mineral density in Crohn's disease: a longitudinal study of budesonide, prednisone and nonsteroid therapy. Am J Gastroenterol. 2002;97:915–21.

34. Stockbrugger RW, Schoon E, Bollani S et al. Budesonide versus prednisolone in the management of Crohn's disease: a randomized multi-national 2-year study. Gastroenterology. 2003;124(Suppl. 1):A26.
35. Leuschner M, Maier KP, Schlichting J et al. Oral budesonide and ursodeoxycholic acid for treatment of primary biliary cirrhosis: results of a prospective double-blind trial. Gastroenterology. 1999;117:918–25.
36. Sandborn WJ, Bengtsson B. Budesonide capsules (Entocort EC) decrease the frequency of psychiatric adverse events compared with prednisolone in Crohn's disease patients: a pooled analysis of 1189 treatment episodes. Gastroenterology. 2002;122 (Suppl. 1):T1664.
37. Lundin PD, Edsbacker S, Bergstrand M et al. Pharmacokinetics of budesonide controlled ileal release capsules in children and adults with active Crohn's disease. Aliment Pharmacol Ther. 2003;17:85–92.
38. Czaja A, Lindor K. Failure of budesonide in a pilot study of treatment-dependent autoimmune hepatitis. Gastroenterology. 2000;119:1312–16.

3
Budesonide in Crohn's disease

V. GROSS

INTRODUCTION

Glucocortoids are the most effective drugs for the treatment of active Crohn's disease. Remission rates of 60–80% may be obtained with conventional systemic glucocorticoids such as prednisone, prednisolone, or 6-methylprednisolone. Because of the high rate of side-effects produced by conventional glucocorticoids budesonide as non-systemic glucocorticoid has been introduced in the treatment of Crohn's disease. Budesonide is a topically active glucocorticoid with a high glucocorticoid receptor affinity and anti-inflammatory potency. Due to its rapid first-pass metabolism and inactivation in the liver, the systemic availability of budesonide is less than 10% after oral dosing. For the treatment of Crohn's disease budesonide has to be administered as an oral retarded preparation in order to avoid its absorption in the upper gastrointestinal tract. Two types of oral budesonide preparation are currently available: a pH-modified release formulation, and a controlled ileal-release formulation. These budesonide preparations have been used to treat active Crohn's disease, to replace systemic glucocorticoids in steroid-dependent patients and to maintain remission of Crohn's disease either induced by glucocorticoids or by surgery.

BUDESONIDE IN ACTIVE CROHN'S DISEASE

A number of randomized controlled trials used oral budesonide in patients with active Crohn's disease. Two trials[1,2] compared budesonide to placebo for the treatment of active Crohn's disease. Five trials[3–7] compared budesonide to conventional systemic glucocorticoids, one trial[8,9] compared budesonide to mesalazine, one trial[10] combined budesonide and antibiotic therapy (Figure 1). Recently a meta-analysis assessing the effectiveness and safety of oral budesonide in comparison to placebo, oral systemic glucocorticoids, and mesalazine has been published[11]. The two studies comparing oral budesonide to placebo found that budesonide induces remission of Crohn's disease more frequently than placebo (RR = 1.85, 95% CI 1.31–2.61). In the study of Greenberg et al.[1] oral doses of 3 mg, 9 mg, and 15 mg of budesonide were compared to placebo in 228 patients with active Crohn's disease. After 8 weeks of treatment, remission was obtained

Study	Plac	BUD 3 mg	BUD 9 mg	BUD 15 mg	Pred
Rutgeerts 1994			53%*		66%
Greenberg 1994	20%	33%*	51%*	43%*	
Campieri 1995			60%*, 42%**		60%
Gross 1996			56%***		73%
Bar-Meir 1998			51%***		53%
Tremaine 2002	33%		48%*, 53%**		

Figure 1 Oral budesonide in active Crohn's disease. Remission rates obtained with budesonide compared to placebo and prednisone/prednisolone in various studies: *, budesonide once daily; **, budesonide b.i.d.; ***, budesonide t.i.d.

in 51% of the patients in the 9 mg budesonide group, in 43% of the patients in the 15 mg group, and in 33% of the patients in the 3 mg group. The remission rate in the placebo group was 20%. Budesonide caused a dose-related reduction in basal and corticotropin-stimulated plasma cortisol concentrations but was not associated with clinically important steroid-related symptoms or other toxic effects. The authors concluded from their study that budesonide at an optimal daily dose of 9 mg is well tolerated and effective against active Crohn's disease in the ileum and proximal colon.

Tremaine et al.[2] treated 200 patients with mild to moderate Crohn's disease either with 9 mg of budesonide once daily, 4.5 mg twice daily, or placebo for 8 weeks. Remission was achieved in 48%, 53%, and 33% with 9 mg budesonide once daily, 4.5 mg twice daily, or placebo, respectively. Differences between the groups were not statistically significant.

In both studies[1,2] total corticosteroid-associated adverse events were not significantly different for patients receiving budesonide compared with patients receiving placebo (50% versus 40%, RR = 1.06, 95% CI 0.92–1.23).

In none of the five trials comparing budesonide to conventional glucocorticoids[3–7] was there a statistically significant difference between the remission rates induced by budesonide or conventional glucocorticoids. However, the meta-analysis[11] showed that conventional glucocorticoids induced remission of Crohn's disease more frequently than budesonide (RR = 0.87, 95% CI 0.76–0.995). In a subgroup analysis of patients with low disease activity, however, budesonide and conventional glucocorticoids induced remission at similar rates (RR = 0.91, 95% CI 0.77–1.07).

Rutgeerts et al.[3] compared budesonide with prednisolone in 176 patients with active ileal or ileocaecal Crohn's disease (88 patients in each group). Budesonide was administered at a dose of 9 mg/day for 8 weeks and then at a dose of 6 mg/day for 2 weeks. Prednisolone was administered at a dose of 40 mg/day for 2 weeks and thereafter was gradually reduced to 5 mg/day. At 10 weeks 53% of the patients in the budesonide group were in remission as compared with 66% of those treated with prednisolone. The mean CDAI decreased from 275 to 175 in the budesonide group and from 279 to 136 in the prednisolone group. Gluco-corticoid-associated side-effects were significantly less in the budesonide group (29 versus 48 patients, $p = 0.003$).

Gross et al.[4] compared 3×3 mg budesonide per day with 6-methylpredniso-lone in patients with active ileal or ileocolonic Crohn's disease. Budesonide induced remission in 55.9% of the patients, 6-methylprednisolone in 72.7% of the patients. This difference was statistically not significant. There was a similar CDAI decrease in both groups (Figure 2). Patients in the budesonide group suffered significantly less frequently from steroid-related side-effects than patients in the 6-methylprednisolone group (28.6% versus 69.7%, $p = 0.0015$).

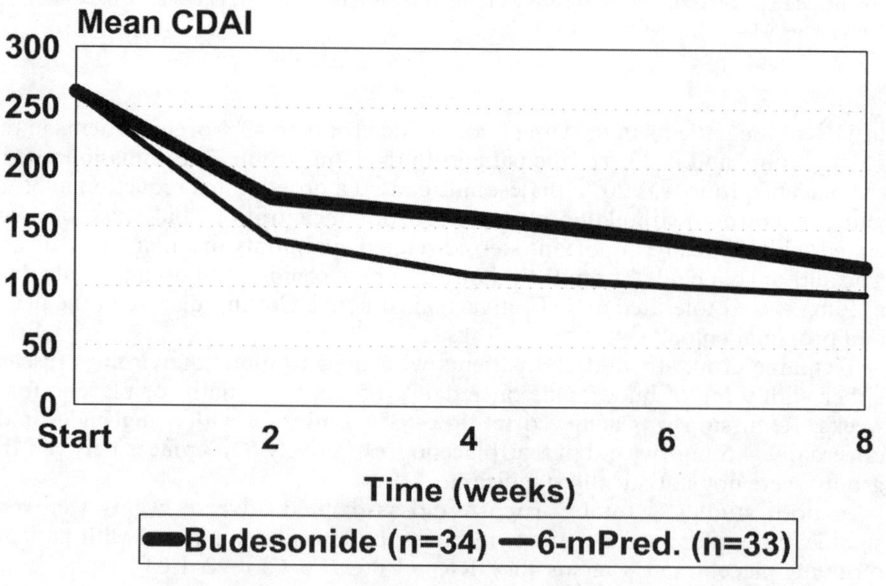

Figure 2 Oral pH-modified release budesonide versus 6-methylprednisolone in active Crohn's disease. Course of CDAI in 34 patients treated with budesonide and in 33 patients treated with 6-methylprednisolone[4]

Campieri et al.[5] compared two regimens of budesonide (1×9 mg and 2×4.5 mg per day) with prednisolone (40 mg starting dose with conventional tapering): 9 mg of budesonide were equally effective as prednisolone, with 60% remission at 8 weeks. The divided dose was somewhat less effective (42%). The suppression of plasma cortisol was much more pronounced in the prednisolone group and was more often severe in the once-daily budesonide group as compared to the divided-dose group.

Bar-Meir et al.[6] compared 3×3 mg budesonide per day with prednisone (starting dose 40 mg/day) in 201 patients with ileocolonic Crohn's disease. Remission rates after 8 weeks were comparably high in the budesonide group (51%) and in the prednisone group (52.5%). However, in the budesonide group twice as many patients reached remission without steroid side-effects (30%) than in the prednisolone group (14%).

The meta-analysis of the studies comparing budesonide to conventional glucocorticoids showed that total glucocorticoid-associated adverse events were significantly less frequent for patients who received budesonide than for patients who received conventional glucocorticoids (RR = 0.65, 95% CI 0.533–0.80)[11]. This means a relative risk reduction of 45%.

The study comparing budesonide to mesalazine[8] showed that budesonide induced remission of Crohn's disease more frequently than mesalazine (62% versus 36%), respectively. This produced a relative risk of 1.73 (95% CI 1.26–2.39). Further analysis of this study showed that budesonide improved health-related quality of life to a greater extent than mesalazine in patients with mild to moderate Crohn's disease[9].

In a recent double-blind multicentre study of patients with active Crohn's disease of the ileum, right colon, or both, patients were randomized to receive 9 mg oral budesonide once daily and in addition oral ciprofloxacin and metronidazole, both 500 mg twice daily, or placebo for 8 weeks. Sixty-six patients received placebo, 64 received antibiotics. At week 8 21 patients (33%) of the antibiotic group achieved remission as compared with 25 patients (38%) of the placebo group (n.s.). Among patients with involvement of the right colon 9/17 (52%) were in remission on the treatment with antibiotics compared with 4/16 (25%) of those who received placebo ($p = 0.15$). Thus, the addition of ciprofloxacin and metronidazole to budesonide was ineffective in patients with active Crohn's disease, but there were some indications that the antibiotic combination may improve the outcome when the colon is involved.

In a further trial[12] oral budesonide was tested in a randomized double-blind dose-finding study (Figure 3). Patients with active Crohn's ileocolitis without steroid pretreatment received either 3×2 mg, 3×3 mg or 3×6 mg budesonide. Remission rates after 6 weeks were 36% (3×2 mg budesonide), 55% (3×3 mg budesonide), and 66% (3×6 mg budesonide) respectively. Only the remission rates of 3×6 mg versus 3×2 mg were significantly different ($p = 0.017$). Patients with high disease activity (CDAI $\geqslant 300$) responded better to the highest budesonide dose (remission rates 0%, 25%, and 75% for 3×2 mg, 3×3 mg, and 3×6 mg budesonide). Steroid-typical side-effects were observed in seven patients (3×2 mg), one patient (3×3 mg), and eight patients (3×6 mg) after 6 weeks of treatment. This study demonstrates that oral pH-modified release budesonide shows a dose-dependent effectiveness in patients with active ileocolonic Crohn's

Remission rate after 6 weeks (%)
70
60
50
40
30
20
10
0
36%*
55%
66%*
6 mg (n=39)
9 mg (n=33)
18 mg (n=32)
*p=0.017 (18 mg vs 6 mg)

A

%
80
60
40
20
0
0%
25%
75%
47%
71%
64%
CDAI >300 (n=25)
CDAI <300 (n=79)
6 mg
9 mg
18 mg

B

%
80
60
40
20
0
30%
60%
59%
31%
46%
73%
Ileum-asc. (n=57)
trans.-rect. (n=44)
6 mg
9 mg
18 mg

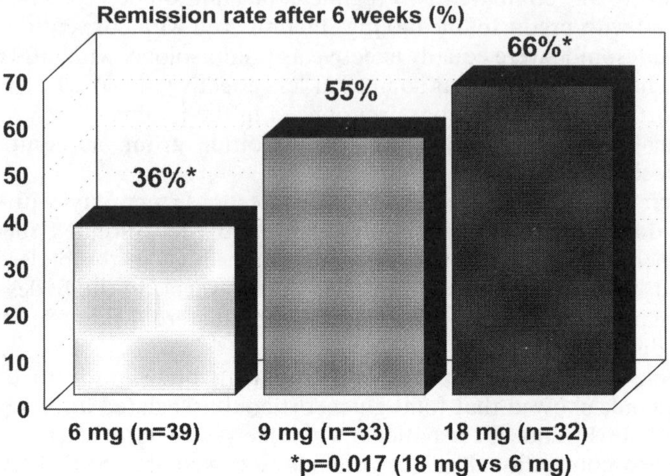

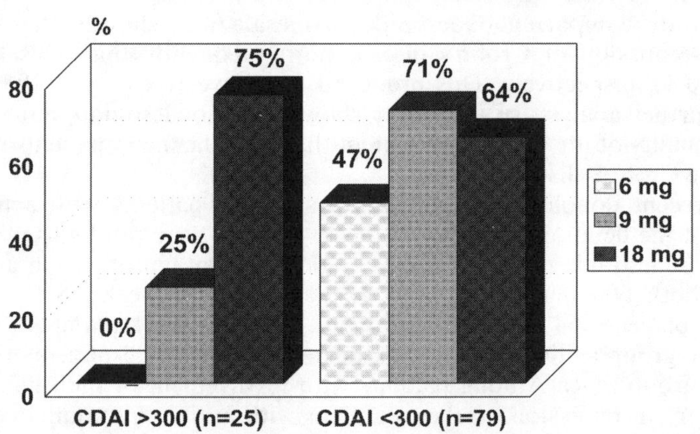

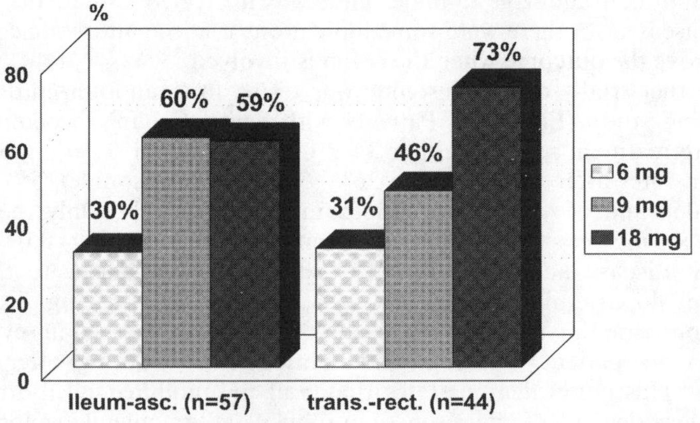

C

disease. In the majority of patients 9 mg budesonide per day are sufficient. In patients with highly active disease higher doses can increase the therapeutic response.

SWITCH FROM SYSTEMIC GLUCOCORTICOIDS TO BUDESONIDE

Two trials assessed the switch from systemic glucocorticoids to budesonide. Cortot et al.[13] evaluated the possibility of switching from systemic glucocorticoids to budesonide in prednisolone/prednisone-dependent patients with inactive Crohn's disease affecting the ileum and/or ascending colon. A total of 120 patients were randomly assigned to receive budesonide 6 mg once daily or placebo. Prednisolone was tapered to zero during the first 4–10 weeks, and budesonide or placebo were given concomitantly and for a further 12 weeks. After 1 and 13 weeks without prednisolone, relapse rates were 17% and 32% in the budesonide group, and 41% and 65% in the placebo group. These differences were statistically significant. The number of glucocorticoid-related side-effects was reduced by 50% by switching from prednisolone to budesonide. The authors conclude from the data that the majority of patients with glucocorticoid-dependent ileocaecal Crohn's disease can be switched to budesonide.

In an open prospective multicentre trial the replacement of conventional glucocorticoids by oral budesonide was studied in patients with active and inactive Crohn's disease[14] (Figure 4). A total of 178 patients with active Crohn's disease ($n = 88$) or Crohn's disease in remission during glucocorticoid treatment ($n = 90$) were included. Conventional glucocorticoids were tapered down during a maximum of 3 weeks with simultaneous intake of 3×3 mg budesonide. Thereafter, patients received 3×3 mg budesonide alone for 6 weeks. The percentage of patients with glucocorticoid-related side-effects decreased from 65.2% at entry to 43.3% at the end of the trial ($p < 0.0001$). The total number of glucocorticoid-related side-effects decreased significantly from 269 to 90; 38.6% of the patients who entered the study with active Crohn's disease under conventional glucocorticoids were in remission at the end of the study. Of the patients who entered the study with Crohn's disease in remission, 78% stayed in remission after switching from conventional glucocorticoids to budesonide.

In conclusion, both studies[13,14] showed that the majority of Crohn's disease patients who are in remission with low doses of prednisone/prednisolone stay in remission when switched to budesonide.

Figure 3 Dose-ranging study with oral pH-modified release budesonide. Patients with active Crohn's ileocolitis were treated either with 6 mg ($n = 39$), 9 mg ($n = 33$) or 18 mg ($n = 32$) of oral pH-modified release budesonide: (**A**) Effect of budesonide dose on overall remission rates. (**B**) Effect of different doses of budesonide in patients with different disease activities. (**C**) Effect of different doses of budesonide in patients with different disease localizations

A

	All patients (n=54)	CDAI <150 (n=24)	CDAI >150 (n=30)
Failure (CDAI >150)	35.2%	8.3%	56.7%
Success (CDAI <150)	63%	91.7%	40%
Drop out (CDAI <150)	1.8%	0%	3.3%

B

	Entry	1. CV (stop of systemic steroid)	4. CV (6 weeks budesonide only)
Patients with side effects	37 (68.5%)	28 (52.8%)	17 (37.8%)
number of side effects	88	47	29
valid n	54	53	45
Mean side effects/patient	1.6	0.9	0.6

Figure 4 Replacement of conventional glucocorticoids by oral pH-modified release budesonide. A total of 178 patients with active Crohn's disease ($n = 88$) or Crohn's disease in remission during glucocorticoid treatment ($n = 90$) were switched to oral pH-modified release budesonide (3×3 mg/day)[14]. The table shows (**A**) remission rates, (**B**) steroid side-effects after 6 weeks of budesonide treatment

BUDESONIDE FOR MAINTENANCE OF REMISSION OF CROHN'S DISEASE

Four trials[15-18] compared budesonide to placebo for the maintenance of glucocorticoid-induced remission of Crohn's disease (Figure 5). Two trials[20,21] tested budesonide compared to placebo for the prevention of postsurgical recurrence in Crohn's disease. Overall, budesonide showed no significant effect on maintaining remission of Crohn's disease more frequently than placebo (RR = 1.08, 95% CI 0.93–1.25). Although 6 mg of budesonide per day significantly prolonged the median time to relapse (158 days versus 39 days in the study of Greenberg et al., 258 days versus 92 days in the study of Löfberg et al.), 6 mg budesonide per day had no statistically significant trend for maintaining remission (RR = 1.13, 95% CI 0.84–1.51). It should be mentioned that in all these studies the 12-month relapse rate of Crohn's disease was rather high. In a further study[19] a fixed (1×6 mg) versus a flexible (3–6 or 9 mg/day) dosing regimen of budesonide was used to maintain remission of Crohn's disease over 12 months. A total of 141 patients with Crohn's disease who had at least one episode of active disease within the preceding 12 months were included in the study. Very low rates of clinical relapses were seen in both treatment groups during 12 months (flexible group 15%, fixed group 19%, $p = 0.61$). The average consumed dose of budesonide was comparable in both groups (5.8 mg in the flexible dosing group, 6.0 mg in the fixed dosing group). Since no placebo group was included in this study it allows no conclusion regarding the efficacy of budesonide.

Hellers et al.[20] found that budesonide did not reduce the overall relapse rate after surgery. Only patients who had been operated for disease activity showed benefit from the prophylactic treatment. Similarly, Ewe et al.[21] found that 3×1 mg of oral budesonide did not reduce the rate of endoscopic and/or clinical relapses within 1 year.

	Placebo	3 mg BUD	6 mg BUD
Loefberg 1996	92d/63%	139d/74%	258d/59%
Greenberg 1996	39d/64%	124d/58%	178d/58%
Gross 1996	67d/65%	94d/67%	
Ferguson 1998	310d/60%	335d/48%	275d/46%

Figure 5 Oral budesonide for maintenance of glucocorticoid-induced remission of Crohn's disease. The table shows median time to relapse (days) and relapse rate after 1 year (%).

CONCLUSION

Budesonide is effective in inducing remission in patients with active Crohn's disease. Budesonide is more likely to induce remission than placebo or mesalazine. Budesonide induces remission less frequently than conventional systemic glucocorticoids (RR = 0.87, 95% CI. 0.76–0.995). In patients with low disease activity (CDAI $\leqslant$ 300) budesonide is as effective as conventional glucocorticoids. Budesonide causes significantly less glucocorticoid-related side-effects than conventional glucocortoids (RR = 0.65, 95% CI 0.53–0.80). Budesonide may be used to replace conventional glucocorticoids in steroid-dependent patients with Crohn's disease. In steroid-dependent patients, however, the use of immunosuppressive agents (azathioprine/6-mercaptopurine) should be considered.

References

1. Greenberg GR, Feagan BG, Martin F et al. and the Canadian Inflammatory Bowel Disease Study Group. Oral budesonide for active Crohn's disease. N Engl J Med. 1994;331:836–41.
2. Tremaine WJ, Hanauer SB, Katz S et al. and the Budesonide CIR United States Study Group. Budesonide CIR capsules (once or twice daily divided-dose) in active Crohn's disease: a randomized placebo-controlled study in the United States. Am J Gastroenterol. 2002;97: 1748–54.
3. Rutgeerts P, Löfberg R, Malchow H et al. A comparison of budesonide with prednisolone for active Crohn's disease. N Engl J Med. 1994;331:842–5.
4. Gross V, Andus T, Caesar I et al. and the German/Austrian Budesonide Study Group. Oral pH-modified release budesonide versus 6-methylprednisolone in active Crohn's disease. Eur J Gastroenterol Hepatol. 1996;8:905–9.
5. Campieri M, Ferguson A, Doe W, Persson T, Nilsson L-G and the Global Budesonide Study Group. Oral budesonide is as effective as oral prednisolone in active Crohn's disease. Gut. 1997;41:209–14.
6. Bar-Meir S, Chowers Y, Lavy A et al. and the Israeli Budesonide Study Group. Budesonide versus prednisone in the treatment of active Crohn's disease. Gastroenterology. 1998;115:835–40.
7. D'Haens G, Verstraete A, Cheyns K et al. Bone turnover during short-term therapy with methylprednisolone or budesonide in Crohn's disease. Aliment Pharmacol Ther. 1998;12:419–24.
8. Thomsen OØ, Cortot A, Jewell D et al. and the International Budesonide-Mesalamine Study Group. A comparison of budesonide and mesalamine for active Crohn's disease. N Engl J Med. 1998;339:370–4.
9. Thomsen OØ, Cortot A, Jewell D et al. for the International Budesonide-Mesalamine Study Group. Budesonide and mesalazine in active Crohn's disease: A comparison of the effects on quality of life. Am J Gastroenterol. 2002;97:649–53.
10. Steinhart AH, Feagan BG, Wong CJ et al. for the Crohn's and Colitis Foundation of Canada Inflammatory Bowel Disease Network Investigators. Combined budesonide and antibiotic therapy for active Crohn's disease: a randomized controlled trial. Gastroenterology. 2002; 123:33–40.
11. Kane SV, Schoenfeld P, Sandborn WJ, Tremaine W, Hofer T, Feagan BG. Systematic review: the effectiveness of budesonide therapy for Crohn's disease. Aliment Pharmacol Ther. 2002; 16:1509–17.
12. Schölmerich J, Gross V, Andus T et al. and the German/Austrian Budesonide Study Group. Dose finding study with oral budesonide in patients with active Crohn's ileocolitis. 2003 (Submitted).
13. Cortot A, Colombel J-F, Rutgeerts P et al. for the International Budesonide Study Group. Switch from systemic steroids to budesonide in steroid dependent patients with inactive Crohn's disease. Gut. 2001;48:186–90.
14. Andus T, Gross V, Caesar I et al. and the German/Austrian Budesonide Study Group. Replacement of conventional glucocorticoids by oral pH-modified release budesonide in

active and inactive Crohn's disease. Results of an open, prospective, multicenter trial. Dig Dis Sci. 2003;48:373–8.

15. Greenberg GR, Feagan BG, Martin F et al. and the Canadian Inflammatory Bowel Disease Study Group. Oral budesonide as maintenance treatment for Crohn's disease: a placebo-controlled, dose-ranging study. Gastroenterology. 1996;110:45–51.

16. Löfberg R, Rutgeerts P, Malchow H et al. Budesonide prolongs time to relapse in ileal and ileocaecal Crohn's disease. A placebo controlled one year study. Gut. 1996;39:82–6.

17. Gross V, Andus T, Ecker KW et al. and the Budesonide Study Group. Low dose oral pH modified release budesonide for maintenance of steroid induced remission in Crohn's disease. Gut. 1998;42:493–6.

18. Ferguson A, Campieri M, Doe W, Persson T, Nygård G and the Global Budesonide Study Group. Oral budesonide as maintenance therapy in Crohn's disease – results of a 12-month study. Aliment Pharmacol Ther. 1998;12:175–83.

19. Green JRB, Lobo AJ, Giaffer M, Travis S, Watkins HC and the Freedom Investigator Group. Maintenance of Crohn's disease over 12 months: fixed versus flexible dosing regimen using budesonide controlled ileal release capsules. Aliment Pharmacol Ther. 2001;15:1331–41.

20. Hellers G, Cortot A, Jewell D et al. and the IOIBD Budesonide Study Group. Oral budesonide for prevention of postsurgical recurrence in Crohn's disease. Gastroenterology. 1999;116:294–300.

21. Ewe K, Böttger T, Buhr HJ, Ecker K-W, Otto HF and the German Budesonide Study Group. Low-dose budesonide treatment for prevention of postoperative recurrence of Crohn's disease: a multicenter randomized placebo-controlled trial. Eur J Gastroenterol Hepatol. 1999;11:277–82

4
Pharmacokinetics after single and multiple oral dosing of budesonide pH-modified-release capsules in patients with distal ulcerative colitis

A. S. PEÑA, J. J. KOLKMAN, R. GREINWALD, H.-D. TAUSCHEL, F. G. NELIS, P. VIERGEVER, A. C. MÖLLMANN, G. HOCHHAUS and H. W. MÖLLMANN

INTRODUCTION

Budesonide has been identified as a suitable topical steroid and is currently used for the treatment of Crohn's disease and ulcerative colitis, given as enteric-coated pellets in gastric juice-soluble capsules or as enemas[1-3]. Gastric juice-soluble hard gelatine capsules, each containing 3 mg budesonide distributed in about 350 gastric juice-resistant pellets with a diameter of about 1 mm for pH-modified release of budesonide (Budenofalk® pH-modified release capsules, PMR) (pH ≥ 6.4) based on the encapsulation of budesonide in methacrylic polymers, has recently been introduced. This delivery form releases the active drug during passage through the ileum and ascending colon, and this has been shown to improve clinical and functional outcomes as quickly and efficiently as systemically acting glucocorticoids such as prednisolone or prednisone in patients with inflammatory bowel diseases[4,5]. Two pilot studies showed that Budenofalk® had a therapeutic effect on the activity of steroid-dependent ulcerative colitis, had a significant steroid-sparing effect, and beneficial effects could be demonstrated by combining the new oral budesonide formulation with budesonide enemas in patients with steroid-dependent ulcerative colitis[6,7]. In an open clinical trial including 72 patients with active ulcerative colitis, it was found that the effects of another formulation of oral budesonide were comparable to prednisolone but, in contrast to prednisolone, budesonide did not change the plasma cortisol level[8].

A case report of a 14-year-old girl suffering from a steroid-dependent chronic active, severe ulcerative colitis demonstrated complete remission after changing from prednisolone to oral Budenofalk® 3 × 3 mg/day, and the progression of osteopenia and growth retardation caused by the prednisolone treatment could be stopped[9].

Previous reports have described the pharmacokinetics and pharmacodynamics of the topically acting budesonide after single and multiple dosage regimens of Budenofalk[®] in healthy volunteers and patients with Crohn's disease, and in ileostomy patients[10].

The aim of the present study was to investigate the clinical efficacy and safety of the topically acting budesonide in patients with mildly to moderately active left-sided ulcerative colitis using the dosage regimens of 3×3 mg or 1×9 mg budesonide per day, to provide pharmacokinetic results on budesonide and its two major metabolites and to assess the budesonide concentrations in biopsy specimens of the rectum, sigmoid and descending colon before treatment and at steady state.

PATIENTS AND METHODS

Fifteen patients with mildly to moderately active proctitis, proctosigmoiditis or left-sided ulcerative colitis were included in the study after diagnosis was confirmed by colonoscopy and histology. The CAI (clinical activity index) score had to be more than 4, and the EI (endoscopic index) score had to be 4 or more[11]. The patients were not allowed to receive any concomitant active medication for ulcerative colitis such as glucocorticoids or an immunosuppressant. In Group A receiving 3×3 mg Budenofalk[®] capsules, the eight patients (six female, two male) with ulcerative colitis included in the evaluation were 30.4 ± 16.54 years old (range 17–67 years), had a body weight of 66.5 ± 13.73 kg (range 48–79 kg) and an average height of 172.9 ± 10.78 cm (range 158–190 cm). In Group B receiving 1×9 mg Budenofalk[®] capsules, the seven patients (four female, three male) with ulcerative colitis included in the evaluation were 48.6 ± 16.38 years old (range 27–69 years), had a body weight of 81.6 ± 17.64 kg (range 56–107 kg) and an average height of 170.6 ± 9.07 cm (range 163–182 cm).

Patients were randomly assigned to receive treatment with either 3×3 mg budesonide per day or 1×9 mg budesonide per day for 8 weeks or for 4 weeks where there was remission after this treatment period, respectively. The patients enrolled in this study were hospitalized on the evening of day 4 for performance of the pharmacokinetic studies (budesonide, 6β-OH-budesonide and 16α-OH-prednisolone concentrations) on day 5, and they stayed until the morning of day 6 for the last blood withdrawal at 7 a.m. In addition, budesonide concentrations were determined in biopsy material of the descending colon (± 50 cm), the sigmoid colon (± 25 cm) and the rectum (± 10 cm) at baseline (day 0) and on day 56 of treatment. The CAI was determined at baseline and after 4 and 8 weeks of treatment in symptomatic patients.

A sensitive, rapid and selective liquid chromatography electrospray ionization tandem mass spectrometry (LC-ESI-MS-MS) method has been developed and validated for the simultaneous quantification of budesonide (BUD) and its major metabolites, 6ß-hydroxybudesonide (6ß-OH-budesonide) and 16α-hydroxyprednisolone (16α-OH-prednisolone) in human plasma.

The pharmacokinetic analysis was performed using non-compartmental approaches using the Kinetica[®] software (version 3.1, InnaPhase Corporation, Philadelphia, PA) which did not differ in pharmacokinetic principles from previously employed Excel® spreadsheets. Data below the limit of detection were not considered, and the following parameters were derived:

1. T_{max} (time of peak concentration) and C_{max}-values (peak concentration) were obtained directly from the concentration vs. time data.

2. The time lag of absorption (t_{lag}) was defined as the time after drug administration at which concentrations increased above baseline values.

3. The area under the concentration–time profile between 0 h (day 5) and the last measurement point after 24 h on day 6 ($AUC_{0-24\ h}$) was calculated by the trapezoidal rule.

4. The terminal elimination rate constant k_e was determined for each individual subject from the terminal slopes of semi-logarithmic plots of serum concentration–time profiles. For the 3×3 mg dosing regimen, generally the time window of 12–24 h was used. The elimination half-life was calculated as $t_{\frac{1}{2}} = 0.693/k_e$.

5. Apparent clearance (Cl) not adjusted for the systemic bioavailability (f) was calculated from $AUC_{0-24\ h}$ and the administered dose ($D = 9$ mg).

6. The clinical efficacy response was defined as $CAI \leqslant 4$ (presence of clinical remission) at day 28 (second control) and day 56 (final control). Non-response was defined as $CAI > 4$ (absence of clinical remission) at the same time. Patients who were not in remission and had discontinued the therapy on day 24 or earlier were considered to be non-responders at both times of assessment.

RESULTS

Only patients with active ulcerative colitis distal to the splenic flexure were included for the assessment of the clinical activity index ($CAI > 4$). After 4 weeks a complete response ($CAI \leqslant 4$) was reached in 0 patients of group A, but in three patients of group B. The overall response rate after 8 weeks ($CAI \leqslant 4$ or decrease CAI 30%) was better with 9 mg o.d. (71%) compared to 3 mg t.i.d. (38%). The endoscopic index (EI) improved from 8.8 ± 2.1 to 3.8 ± 4.7 ($p = 0.02$) in 3 mg t.i.d. and from 9.7 ± 2.1 to 2.0 ± 2.9 ($p < 0.001$) in 9 mg o.d.

Mean budesonide and 6β-OH-budesonide serum profiles were markedly different between treatment groups, with higher peak concentrations obtained following the single 9 mg dose compared to the more sustained drug profile obtained when the same dose was administered in three divided portions at 5 h intervals as shown in Figure 1. The similar profiles for budesonide and 6β-OH-budesonide, in conjunction with higher levels of 16α-OH-prednisolone and a lag-time of about 3 h, are consistent with prolonged absorption of drug.

Concentrations measured in biopsy specimens obtained on day 0 and day 56 of the clinical trial showed increased budesonide levels after treatment, with no distinct differences between regional concentrations and dosing regimens, when the distinct variability in the concentrations is considered (results not shown).

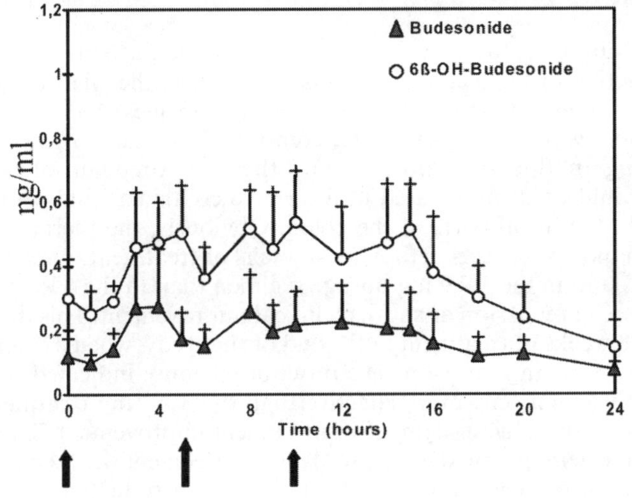

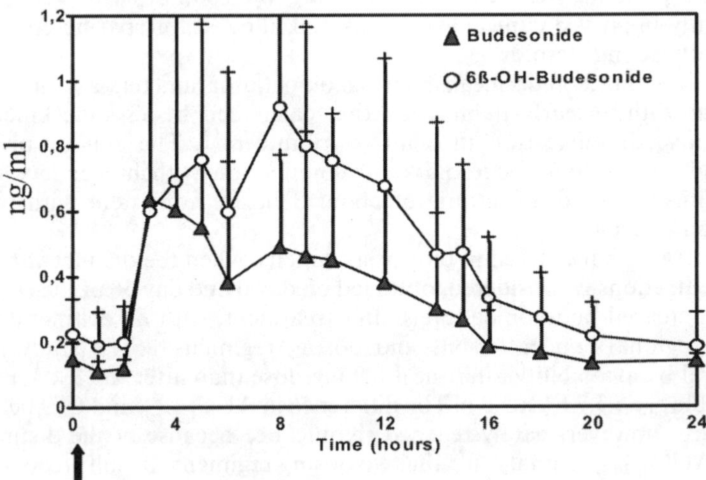

Figure 1 Mean serum budesonide and 6β-OH-budesonide ($\pm$SD) on day 5 of dosing in patients with left-sided ulcerative colitis. Group A (above): 3 mg budesonide oral capsules three times daily at 0, 5 and 10 h as indicated by arrows; group B (below) 9 mg budesonide as oral controlled-release capsules at 0 h

DISCUSSION

The present clinical study on oral budesonide in patients with mildly to moderately active distal ulcerative colitis shows that the pH-modified release formulation of budesonide (Budenofalk® 3 mg capsules) induces a treatment effect in about two-thirds of patients, comparable to that of mesalazine, the standard drug in this indication[12]. For the first time an efficacy of oral budesonide could be demonstrated in ulcerative colitis patients with inflammation limited to the distal parts of the colon. Obviously, the therapeutic effect is dependent on the dosage regimen. After 4 weeks of treatment, remarkably better results were found in the 1×9 mg dosage regimen than in the 3×3 mg regimen: 57% vs 0% were in remission or showed clinical improvement. This difference was smaller after 8 weeks of treatment at the end of the study, when 57% (group B) vs 38% (group A) were in remission. The onset of response indicated that the 1×9 mg treatment was not only more effective than the 3×3 mg treatment, but was also much faster in inducing remission or clinical improvement. The efficacy of oral budesonide demonstrated in this study is in agreement with the results of two earlier trials in ulcerative colitis as indicated in the introduction. Another study on oral budesonide in ulcerative colitis investigated the efficacy and safety of the pH-modified release formulation (Budenofalk® 3 mg capsules) in steroid-dependent patients. A daily dose of 9 mg budesonide was well tolerated, significantly improved clinical symptoms and allowed for sparing conventional, systemically acting steroids[13].

Results for budesonide mean pharmacokinetic parameters are in reasonable agreement with an early publication that calculated budesonide kinetics after intravenous administration in healthy volunteers[14]. The similar profiles for budesonide and 6β-OH-budesonide, in conjunction with higher levels of 16α-OH-prednisolone and a lag-time of about 3 h, are consistent with prolonged absorption of drug.

Concentrations measured in biopsy specimens, when the distinct variability in the concentrations is considered, obtained on day 0 and day 56 of the clinical trial showed increased budesonide levels after treatment, with no distinct differences between regional concentrations and dosing regimens[15]. The study indicated higher oral bioavailability after the 1×9 mg dose than after the 3×3 mg dose at comparable t_{max}: 5.7 h vs. 5.3 h. The difference in $AUC_{0-24\,h}$ and Cl/f between the two groups, however, barely reached significance because of the distinct variability in $AUC_{0-24\,h}$ estimates for the two dosing regimens. Results from this study indicate that higher peak concentrations of parent drug and metabolites are obtained when a single 9 mg dose of budesonide is administered as controlled-release capsules compared to administration of 9 mg in three divided doses over 10 h. Although the data suggest increased total absorption of drug with a single administration, AUC values were not significantly different due to the high variability between patients with ulcerative colitis[15].

The study also assessed the drug levels in biopsy specimens after 56 days of treatment. Considering the limited amount of data, and the distinct variability, it is difficult to assess whether regional differences in the budesonide content between descending and sigmoid colon or rectum exist.

Since all patients in this study suffered from inflammation limited to the left-sided colon and/or rectum, and the pharmacokinetic investigations demonstrated therapeutically adequate mucosal budesonide concentrations in these regions, it can be concluded that the active drug from both dosage regimens of Budenofalk® 3 mg capsules used in this study is effective in the whole colon, even reaching far distal gut regions. The good tolerability profile without serious drug-related adverse events as compared to the conventional, systemically acting steroids suggests that this topically acting, pH-modified release formulation of budesonide could be a treatment option in active ulcerative colitis.

References

1. Campieri M. New steroids and new salicylates in inflammatory bowel disease: a critical appraisal. Gut. 2002;50(Suppl. 3):iii43–6.
2. Kane SV, Schoenfeld P, Sandborn WJ, Tremain W, Hofer T, Feagan BG. Systemic review: the effectiveness of budesonide therapy for Crohn's disease. Aliment Pharmacol Ther. 2002;16: 1509–17.
3. Sandborn WJ, Feagan BG. Review article: Mild to moderate Crohn's disease – defining the basis for a new treatment algorithm. Aliment Pharmacol Ther. 2003;18:263–77.
4. Rutgeerts P, Löfberg R, Malchow H et al. A comparison of budesonide with prednisolone for active Crohn's disease. N Engl J Med. 1994;331:842–5.
5. Bar-Meir S, Chowers Y, Lavy A et al. Budesonide versus prednisone in the treatment of active Crohn's diesease. Gastroenterology. 1998;115:835–40.
6. Deusch K, Mauthe B, Spießl G, Classen M. Budesonide in the treatment of steroid dependent inflammatory bowel disease (abstract 29). Falk Symposium No. 72: IV. Internationales Symposium über chronisch entzündliche Darmerkrankungen, 6–8 September 1993, Strasbourg, France.
7. Köhne G. Budesonide in the treatment of steroid dependent ulcerative pancolitis. Abstracts II (Poster presentations) 178P. World Congresses of Gastroenterology, 2–7 October, 1993, Los Angeles, USA.
8. Löfberg R, Danielsson Å, Nilsson A et al. Oral budesonide versus prednisolone in patients with active extensive and left-sided ulcerative colitis. Gastroenterology. 1996;110:1713–18.
9. Hüppe D, Schenck B, Tromm A, Bürk G. Budesonide treatment in a 14-year old girl with chronic active ulcerative colitis (abstract 51). Falk Symposium No. 72. IV. Internationales Symposium über entzündliche Darmerkrankungen, 6–8 September, 1993, Strasbourg, France.
10. Möllmann HW, Hochhaus G, Tromm A et al. Pharmacokinetics and pharmacodynamics of budesonide-pH-modified release capsules. In: Möllmann HW, May B, editors. Glucocorticoid Therapy in Chronic Inflammatory Bowel Disease – From Basic Principles to Rational Therapy. Dordrecht: Kluwer, 1996:107–20.
11. Rachmilewitz D (on behalf of an international Study group). Coated mesalazine (5-aminosalicylic acid) vs. sulphasalazine in the treatment of active ulcerative colitis: a randomised trial. Br Med J. 1989;298:82–6.
12. Schroeder KW. Role of mesalazine in acute and long-term treatment of ulcerative colits and its complications. Scand J Gastroenterol. 2002;37(Suppl. 236):42–7.
13. Keller R, Stoll R, Foerster EC, Gutsche N, Domschke W. Oral budesonide therapy for steroid-dependent ulcerative colitis: a pilot trial. Aliment Pharmacol Ther. 1997;11:1047–52.
14. Ryrfeldt A, Andersson P, Edsbacker S, Tonnesson M, Davies D, Pauwels R. Pharmacokinetics and metabolism of budesonide, a selective glucocorticoid, Eur J Respir Dis Suppl. 1982;122:86–95.
15. Kolkman JJ, Möllmann HW, Hochhaus G et al. Clinical and pharmacological comparison of oral budesonide 3×1 mg vs. 1×9 mg per day in patients with active distal ulcerative colitis. (In preparation).

Section II
Potential use of budesonide in inflammatory bowel disease

5
Potential use of budesonide in inflammatory bowel diseases: extended ulcerative colitis

R. KELLER

INTRODUCTION

Glucocorticosteroids (GCS) are the most effective drugs for the treatment of ulcerative colitis (UC)[1,2]. They have a broad spectrum of anti-inflammatory and immunosuppressive actions[3,4], but may also exert significant systemic side-effects[5]. The most serious side-effects, some of which are irreversible, are associated with long-term treatment. In some cases of Crohn's disease (CD) and UC, reduction or cessation of conventional GCS (c-GCS) treatment leads to relapse.

Budesonide is part of a separate class of GCS. It has a high topical anti-inflammatory effect due to its high affinity for the GCS receptor and low systematic availability by virtue of its extensive first-pass hepatic metabolism with resultant metabolites virtually devoid of significant GCS activity. Budesonide has been used in the treatment of asthma, obstructive pulmonary diseases and in Crohn's disease in an oral formulation designed to be released in the ileum and proximal colon with efficacy similar to that of conventional steriods, but with few adverse events and significantly less impact on the hypothalamic–pituitary–adrenal axis. An enema formulation has been designed to deliver the drug to the distal colon in left-sided UC[6,7].

TARGETED DRUG DELIVERY SYSTEMS

In addition to the use of topically acting steroids two decisive principles are necessary to reduce the adverse effects of steroid therapy of UC: a topical drug delivery system with a colon-targeted preparation. There are several approaches for delivering drugs to the large intestine[8–11]; these approaches include pH-controlled delivery designed to release drugs in the more alkaline environment of the lower gastrointestinal tract, enzyme-controlled delivery based on existing enzyme-producing microorganisms in the large intestine, time-controlled delivery with a lag time for onset of release which has to cover transit through the stomach and the small intestine and a pressure-controlled delivery.

The pH value of normal subjects in the terminal ileum has been measured at 7.5 ± 0.4. There is a drop in pH to a mean of 6.4 ± 0.4 in the caecum and then the pH remains between 6.4 and 7.0 from the ascending colon to the left colon. Mucosal pH in the colon tends to be higher than luminal pH, but the luminal pH in patients with IBD can be lower than that measured in normal volunteers[11].

For delivery in the large intestine coated pellets are needed, being resistant against gastric acid with a drug-releasing delay for the small bowel. Multiple unit preparations are the appropriate formulation for delivery in the large intestine compared to single-unit preparations.

BUDESONIDE IN ORAL FORMULATIONS

At present two types of oral budesonide are available: controlled-ileal release capsules and a pH-modified release formulation. Both formulations have been evaluated and were used in the therapy of Crohn's disease. The controlled-ileal release formulation is composed of hard gelatin capsules, acid-resistant pellets Eudragit L 100-55, and has a delayed release at pH >5.5. The pH-modified release formulation is also composed of gelatin capsules and acid-resistant pellets. In contrast with the controlled-ileal release formulation the pH-modified release formulation consists of a composition of Eudragit L, S, LS, and RS, and it has a delayed release at pH >6.4.

CLINICAL STUDIES WITH ORAL BUDESONIDE

In 1996 Löfberg et al. published their experience with an oral formulation of budesonide for the treatment of moderately active UC[12]. This study was of randomized, double-blind, double-dummy design with two parallel groups, and the total treatment time was 9 weeks. A total of 72 patients were treated with budesonide or prednisolone, 34 patients received budesonide and 38 patients received prednisolone. Budesonide was administered in a dose of 10 mg, 6 mg in the morning and 4 mg in the evening, during 4 weeks and was tapered to 4 mg once daily in treatment week 9. Prednisolone was administered in a single morning dose of 40 mg and was reduced to 5 mg daily in treatment week 9. The mean endoscopic scores decreased with time significantly in both groups. When the scores were analysed separately for each of the five colorectal segments (ascending colon, transverse colon, descending colon, sigmoid colon, and rectum), a significantly greater improvement was observed in the sigmoid colon for the prednisolone group after 4 weeks. There were no significant differences in the endoscopic scores between patients with extensive or left-sided UC. The histopathological scores were significantly reduced compared with baseline in both groups. The reduction in histopathological scores was significantly greater in the prednisolone group. A separate analysis for each of the colorectal segments showed that the better effect of prednisolone was limited to the descending and sigmoid colon, where a significant difference was found at 4 weeks.

This study has shown that the topically active glucocorticosteroid budesonide, administered in an oral controlled release formulation at an initial dose of 10 mg/day, seems to give an overall treatment result in patients with active UC, approaching that of 40 mg/day of prednisolone with gradual tapering, but without any suppression of morning plasma cortisol levels. Because endoscopic and histological improvement in the distal colon occured preferential in cases treated with prednisolone, this could indicate a suboptimal release of budesonide in this region.

PATIENTS AND METHODS

In our study, 14 inpatients and outpatients (three females, 11 males; mean age 38.1 years, range 18–66 years) with an established diagnosis of UC were eligible for treatment[13]. All patients gave their written informed consent to participate. They were treated on a compassionate use basis. The patients had a minimum of 1 year continuous steroid-dependent UC. During the 1 year prior to this pilot study they recieved c-GCS dependent of the activity of the disease. In cases of high activity they were initially treated with 1 mg prednisolone-equivalent per kilogram body weight daily. In addition, some had more than one relapse within 1 year brought on by reduction of c-GCS. This development was defined as 'steroid-dependent'. The decision whether c-GCS could not be reduced down was made by the doctor who was the study doctor. The patient's opinion was no reason for continuing or finishing c-GCS therapy. The protocols used for reducing c-GCS before and after the introduction of budesonide were similiar (reduction in steps of 5–10 mg prednisolone-equivalent per week).

In all patients the extension and level of activity of disease were verified via routine colonoscopy during the 6 months prior to the beginning of treatment. The patients received budesonide in a pH-modified formulation (Budenofalk®) in a dose of 9 mg (3 × 3 mg) daily of budesonide at stage 10–20 mg prednisolone-equivalent daily and at CAI level lower than 8. After carrying out c-GCS and budesonide therapy simultaneously for 1 week, c-GCS was reduced to 0 mg in steps of 5–10 mg per week. Patients were then treated for at least 6 months with budesonide alone, but therapy was discontinued if the patient's condition deteriorated significantly.

RESULTS

All patients had already been treated with c-GCS for at least 1 year. During the year preceding budesonide treatment, c-GCS therapy could only briefly be terminated in 10 cases (71%), and in four cases (29%) it was not possible to suspend c-GCS therapy at all (see Figure 1). The average c-GCS dosage during the pre-budesonide period was approximately 20 mg prednisolone-equivalent daily. At the conclusion of this 12-month period the average dose of c-GCS was reduced to 15 mg prednisolone-equivalent daily, and budesonide therapy consisting of 9 mg daily (3 × 3 mg) was begun.

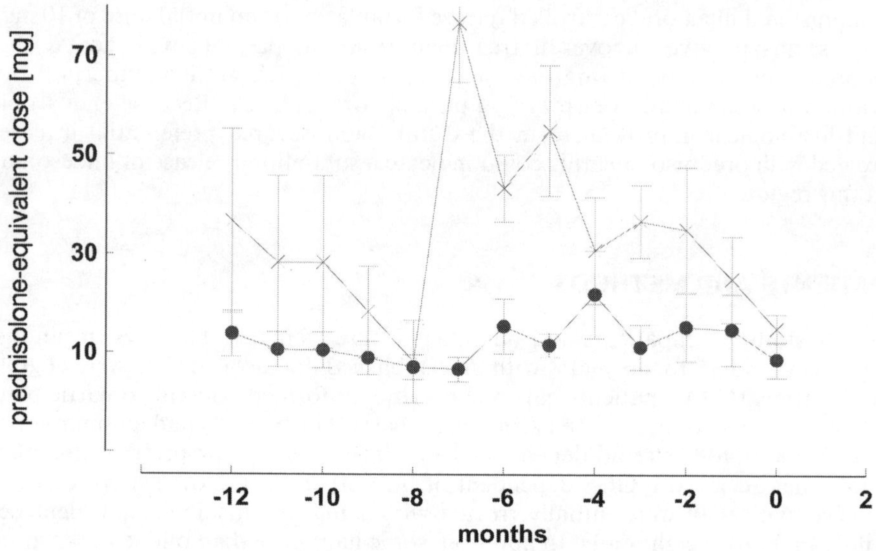

Figure 1 Mean dose of prednisolone-equivalents in the remission group patients (●) and relapse group patients (×) with SEM during the 1 year prior to budesonide treatment

Table 1 Characteristics of budesonide-treated patients with remission or relapse

	Remission group	*Relapse group*	*Both groups*
Patients	11	3	14
Sex (male/female)	8/3	3/0	11/3
Mean age (years, range)	38.7 (18–66)	35.7 (30–43)	38.1 (18–66)
Mean disease duration (years, range)	8 (2–21)	5 (4–6)	7.4 (2–21)
Mean CAI before budesonide treatment	4.7	7.4	5.3
Mean CAI at the beginning of budesonide treatment	2.5	4.7	3
Mean daily prednisolone dose before budesonide treatment (mg)	16.9	30.7	19.9

During the following 6 months, three patients on budesonide (relapse group, 21.4%; Table 1) had a relapse with a CAI of more than 8. Relapse was seen after 1 month in one patient, after 2 months in another patient and after 3 months in a third. Remission was achieved in 11 patients (remission group, 78.6%; Table 1).

In relapse group patients the average dose of prednisolone-equivalent over the year before treatment with budesonide had been 30.7 mg daily as compared to 16.9 mg daily in the remission group patients; the mean CAI of relapse group patients had been 7.4 and of remission group patients 4.7 before commencement of budesonide. These latter differences were statistically significant while CAI differences were not, at the beginning of budesonide treatment (4.7 vs 2.5; $p = 0.191$).

In the remission group patients the CAI dropped significantly upon treatment with budesonide (see Figure 2). Consequently, in all patients of this group prednisolone therapy could be terminated within 3 months of beginning budesonide treatment.

Within the 6-month period of budesonide therapy improvements in ESR, leucocyte count, platelets, C-reactive protein and serum orsomucoid were observed, and no other clinically relevant changes in haematology or clinical chemistry were noted. Mean pulse rate and blood pressure were unchanged. No corticosteroid-associated side-effects were seen. Plasma cortisol value and corticotropin hormone stimulation tests were not carried out. No other side-effects were noted during treatment with budesonide.

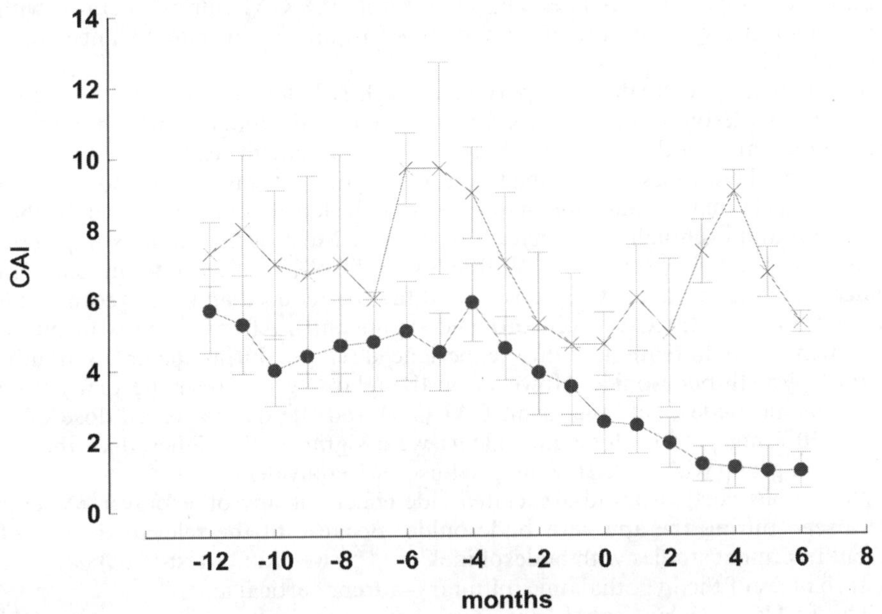

Figure 2   Mean ulcerative colitis clinical activity index (CAI) in the remission group patients (●) and relapse group patients (×) with SEM. The CAI was assessed every month during treatment with prednisolone-equivalents and during treatment with budesonide. The CAI in the remission group could be reduced significantly ($p = 0.00016$)

DISCUSSION

In relapse-prevention studies budesonide 6 mg daily was used to maintain remission in CD[14,15]. These studies showed that this topically acting GCS prolongs the asymptomatic stage in patients with ileal or ileocaecal CD[15]. However, during follow-up it was found that relapse occurred after 1 year of treatment with 6 mg budesonide daily[16].

Oral budesonide treatment was also shown to be effective in the induction of remission in patients with active UC[17].

It was the above-mentioned positive results of treatment of CD and of active UC with budesonide[16] that led us to carry out maintenance treatment of 14 patients with steroid-dependent UC using budesonide 9 mg daily. For this treatment we used a dosage regime of 3 mg budesonide three times daily in a pH-modified formulation[17]. This formulation of oral budesonide (Budenofalk, Dr Falk Pharma, Freiburg, Germany) is very similiar to a formulation of 5-aminosalicylic acid (5-ASA) (Salofalk, Dr Falk Pharma, Freiburg, Germany). The results of a study by Goebell et al.[18] demonstrate that most of the 5-ASA from this slow-release preparation is delivered into the colon, which explains its effectiveness in UC. Therefore a therapy of UC with this formulation of oral budesonide might be possible. The changes in the CAI during therapy with budesonide demonstrate the efficacy of this formulation in maintenance treatment of UC.

The patients we treated are part of a 'high-risk for relapse' group. Before beginning budesonide therapy, c-GCS treatment had brought about remission; during reduction of the daily c-GCS dose, however, patients experienced relapse. In most of these cases a combined administration of 9 mg budesonide and an average of 15 mg prednisolone-equivalent daily led to uncomplicated further reduction and eventually termination of c-GCS. Most of the patients improved with respect to bowel symptoms. Within 3 months of initiation of treatment with budesonide the average c-GCS dose could first be reduced and then terminated, and within 6 months CAI levels dropped significantly. After 6 months 11 out of 14 patients were in remission; three experienced relapse during the first 3 months of therapy with budesonide. However, in the relapse group over the year before commencing budesonide the mean CAI (7.4) and the daily average dose of c-GCS (30.7 mg prednisolone-equivalent) were significantly higher than that in remission group (CAI 4.7; 16.9 mg prednisolone-equivalent).

No serious corticosteroid-associated side-effects or any other adverse events were seen during therapy with budesonide. Because of the relevant results of recent treatment studies with budesonide[14,15,19–21] we did not test specifically for disturbances of the hypothalamic–pituitary–adrenocortical axis.

The 14 UC cases presented here show that the topically acting corticosteroid budesonide, given in an oral pH-modified release formulation at a daily dosage of 9 mg (3×3 mg), significantly reduces CAI. In most cases therapy with c-GCS could be terminated and the time to relapse after c-GCS-induced remission could be prolonged. In our study budesonide was well tolerated without occurrence of serious corticosteroid-associated side-effects.

FURTHER APPROACHES

A number of drug delivery approaches have been advocated. The prodrug approach is a unique method used to carry and release certain corticosteroids to the large intestine[22]. By utilizing the C_{21} hydroxyl group a variety of glycoside prodrugs can be easily synthesized. Being larger and more polar than parent drug, glycoside derivatives of corticosteroids are poorly absorbed from the gastrointestinal tract. This approach to colonic delivery has been explored in a number of studies with prodrugs of different corticosteroids. Nolen et al. treated male Sprague-Dawley rats after induction of an acetic acid-induced pancolitis with intragastric infusion of two prodrugs, dexamethasone-β-D glucuronide (DXglrd) and budesonide-β-D glucuronide (BUDglrd). Tissue levels of DX in healthy rats were high, suggesting an affinity of the large intestine mucosa for DX. These levels increased when DX was dosed as its prodrug. The highest concentration of budesonide was found in the mucosa of the healthy rats following administration of BUDglrd. In colitic rats luminal levels of budesonide were decreased in the caecum compared with that in healthy rats

Rodriguez et al. tested a microparticulate system containing budesonide, in the treatment of TNBS-induced colitis in male Sprague-Dawley rats[23]. The therapeutic effects of budesonide when administered in this system were compared with those obtained after the administration of drug alone, or the drug included in simple enteric microparticles. Macroscopic and histological damage indices were lowest in rats dosed with the new budesonide-loaded microparticulate system; therefore the administration of this new microparticulate system may represent an effective tool for the treatment of human colonic inflammatory bowel disease. This new colonic delivery system significantly improved the efficacy of budesonide in the healing of induced colitis in rats. There were no significant differences, however, when the new treatment was compared with the control formulation consisting of simple enteric microparticles.

CONCLUSIONS

Budesonide plays an important role in the treatment of UC by virtue of its high topical anti-inflammatory and low systemic availability with few adverse events. The delivery of budesonide from microencapsulated cellulosic cores shows no significant differences compared with the control formulation of simple enteric microparticles containing compositions of Eudragit. There are no significant differences between budesonide-prodrug and budesonide in local effects at the colonic mucosa of UC patients. Budesonide in an oral pH-modified release formulation reduces CAI and dosage of c-GCS in patients suffering from extended UC.

References

1. Truelove SC, Witts LJ. Cortisone in ulcerative colitis. Final report on a therapeutical trial. Br Med J. 1955;2:1041–8.
2. Kjeldsen J. Treatment of ulcerative colitis with high doses of oral prednisolone. The rate of remission, the need for surgery, and the effect of prolonging the treatment. Scand J Gastroenterol. 1993;28:821–6.
3. Manso G, Baker A, Taylor I, Fuller R. *In vivo* and *in vitro* effects of glucocorticosteroids on arachidonic acid metabolism and monocyte function in nonasthmatic humans. Eur Respir J. 1992;5:712–16.
4. Linden M. The effects of β2-adrenoceptor agonists and a corticosteroid, budesonide, on the secretion of inflammatory mediators from monocytes. Br J Pharmacol. 1992;107:156–60.
5. Kusunoki M, Möeslein G, Shoji Y et al. Steroid complications in patients with ulcerative colitis. Dis Colon Rectum. 1992;35:1003–9.

6. Lindgren S, Löfberg R, Bergholm L et al. Effect of budesonide enema on remission and relapse rate in distal ulcerative colitis and proctitis. Scand J Gastroenterol. 2002;37:705–10.

7. Hanauer SB, Robinson M, Pruitt R et al. Budesonide enema for the treatment of active, distal ulcerative colitis and proctitis. Gastroenterology. 1998;115:525–32.

8. Rubinstein A. Approaches and opportunities in colon-specific drug delivery. Crit Rev Ther Drug Carrier Syst. 1995;12:101–49.

9. Friend DR. Colon-specific drug delivery. Adv Drug Del Rev. 1991;7:149–99.

10. Rubinstein A. Microbially controlled drug delivery to the colon. Biopharm Drug Dispos. 1990;11:465–75.

11. Friend DR. Issues in oral administration of locally acting glucocorticosteroids for treatment of inflammatory bowel disease. Aliment Pharmacol Ther. 1998;12:591–603.

12. Löfberg R, Daniellson Å, Suhr O et al. Oral budesonide versus prednisolone in patients with active extensive and left-sided ulcerative colitis. Gastroenterology. 1996;110:1713–8.

13. Keller R, Stoll R, Foerster EC, Gutsche N, Domschke W. Oral budesonide therapy for steroid-dependent ulcerative colitis: a pilot trial. Aliment Pharmacol Ther. 1997;11:1047–52.

14. Edsbäcker S, Wollmer P, Nilsson A, Nilsson M. Pharmacokinetics and gastrointestinal transit of budesonide controlled ileal release (CIR) capsules. Gastroenterology. 1993;104 (Suppl.): A695 (abstract).

15. Greenberg G, Feagan B, Martin F et al. and the Canadian Inflammatory Bowel Disease Study Group. Oral budesonide for the treatment of active Crohn's disease. N Engl J Med. 1994;331: 836–41.

16. Löfberg R, Rutgeerts P, Malchow H et al. Budesonide prolongs time to relapse in ileal and ileocaecal Crohn's disease. A placebo controlled one year study. Gut. 1996;39:82–6.

17. Möllmann HW, Hochhaus G, Tromm A et al. Pharmacokinetics and pharmacodynamics of budesonide pH-modified release capsules. In: Möllmann HW, May B, editors. Glucocorticoid Therapy in Chronic Inflammatory Bowel Disease. Dordrecht: Kluwer, 1996:107–20.

18. Goebell H, Klotz U, Nehlsen B, Layer P. Oroileal transit of slow release 5-aminosalicylic acid. Gut. 1993;34:669–75.

19. Greenberg, GR, Feagan BG, Martin F et al. and the Canadian Inflammatory Bowel Disease Study Group. Oral budesonide as maintenance treatment for Crohn's disease: a placebo-controlled, dose-ranging study. Gastroenterology. 1996;110:45–51.

20. Löfberg R, Rutgeerts P, Malchow H et al. Budesonide prolongs time to relapse in ileal and ileocaecal Crohn's disease. A placebo controlled one year study. Gut. 1996;39:82–6.

21. Roth M, Gross V, Schölmerich J, Ueberschaer B, Ewe K. Treatment of active Crohn's disease with an oral slow-release budesonide formulation. Am J Gastroenterol. 1993;88:968–9.

22. Nolen HW, Fedorak RN, Friend DR. Steady-state pharmacokinetics of corticosteroid delivery from glucuronide produgs in normal and colitic rats. Biopharm Drug Dispos. 1997; 18:681–95.

23. Rodriguez M, Antunez JA, Taboada C, Seijo B, Torres D. Colon-specific delivery of budesonide from microencapsulated cellulosic cores: evaluation of the efficacy against colonic inflammation in rats. J Pharm Pharmacol. 1999;51:1107–12.

6
The role of budesonide in the treatment of collagenous and lymphocytic colitis

F. BAERT

INTRODUCTION

What are the clinical criteria for diagnosis of collagenous and lymphocytic colitis?

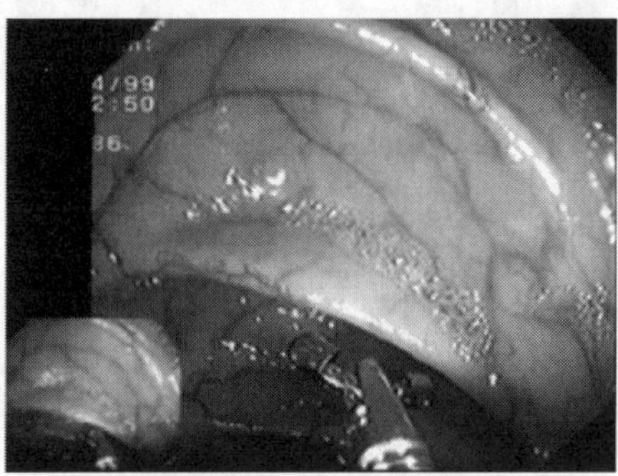

Figure 1 The diagnosis relies on colonic biopsies from macroscopic normal mucosa

Note: The term 'microscopic colitis' is confusing as it is both used as a former name of lymphocytic colitis and as general name for both entities. Therefore in recent publications most authors agree that this term should no longer be used.

1. Chronic watery diarrhoea.

2. Negative stool exam (culture, parasites, and *Clostridium difficile* toxin)

3. Other obvious reasons for diarrhoea should be excluded (e.g. Crohn's disease, ulcerative colitis, lactose intolerance, irritable bowel syndrome, etc.).

4. Associated with autoimmune disease in about 30–40% of cases.

5. Frequently associated with coeliac disease* (no effect of gluten-free diet on biopsies or symptoms).

What are the endoscopic criteria for diagnosis of collagenous and lymphocytic colitis?

Full (ileo)colonoscopy shows no signs of macroscopic inflammation or any other significant findings (e.g. tumour or polyp) (sometimes slight oedema may occur). Random biopsies from different segments of the colon should be obtained.

What is the patient age and sex profile of the two entities?

Collagenous, 75–80% females; lymphocytic, 60% females; average age at diagnosis is 65 (but can occur from the age of 20 on).

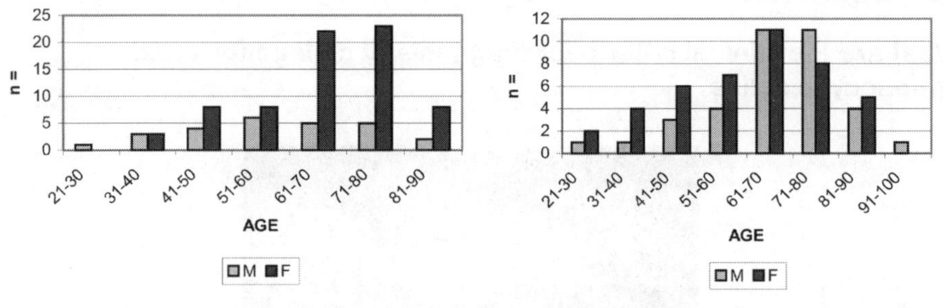

a   b

Figure 2 (a) Age and sex distribution of a large group of collagenous colitis patients; (b) age and sex distribution of a large group of lymphocytic colitis patients

WHAT DO THE BIOPSIES SHOW? ARE COLLAGENOUS COLITIS AND LYMPHOCYTIC COLITIS DIFFERENT ENTITIES?

Histological criteria

The diagnosis of collagenous and lymphocytic colitis is based on a characteristic picture of the colonic mucosal biopsies. The colonoscopy should be macroscopically normal (or near-normal) and biopsies should not be taken in the vicinity of a tumour or significant polyp. All biopsies obtained from different segments should show the same findings, although there may be some regional differences.

---

*Patients with coeliac disease with persistent diarrhoea and strictly adhering to their gluten-free diet should undergo a full colonoscopy with colonic biopsies to look for signs of collagenous colitis and especially of lymphocytic colitis.

Although the diagnostic criteria are clear and stringent, they can easily be overlooked. Clinicians should ask their pathologist specifically to look for the collagen band and for the presence of intra-epithelial lymphocytes. Both common and specific histological criteria for both entities are given in Table 1. Collagenous colitis and lymphocytic colitis are related, but different, clinical and histological entities. Overlap forms occur in about 25%.

Table 1   Histologic criteria for collagenous and lymphocytic colitis

---

Common criteria exist for both conditions
1.   Mixed inflammatory infiltrate in the lamina propria.

2.   Mild regenerative epithelial changes often present including mucin depletion, surface epithelial damage and sloughing, rare infiltration of neutrophils or eosinophils.

Specific criteria include
For collagenous colitis
Average thickness* of a subepithelial collagen band more than 10 μm with a typical feathery-shaped appearance of the inferior margin.

For lymphocytic colitis
The number of intraepithelial lymphocytes is >20 per 100 epithelial cells.

---

*Measurements of the collagen band should be performed on a well-oriented section of the mucosa showing at least three adjacent crypts cut in the same vertical plane.

AETIOLOGY AND PATHOGENESIS

Pathophysiology: hypothesis and arguments

Both collagenous and lymphocytic colitis are idiopathic inflammatory conditions causing inflammation confined to the colonic mucosa. A precise pathophysiological mechanism cannot be proposed, but experimental and epidemiological observations can shed some light on the pathogenesis.

The current evidence suggests that both entities are related, but distinct syndromes triggered by luminal antigens, perpetuated by shared antigens and mediated by cytokines and leukotrienes.

Arguments for putative luminal antigens

1. The histological changes and nature of the lamina propria infiltrate (namely the CD4$^+$ T cells) suggest a processed exogenous antigen.

2. In patients with diverticulosis the histological changes cannot be found within the diverticuli.

3. Surgical ileostomies (hereby diverting the entire colon from the faecal stream) performed in refractory cases improve the symptoms with disappearance of the collagen band.

4. Striking similarities (and frequent) associations with coeliac disease (see below).

5. Oral drugs causing collagenous and lymphocytic colitis (see below).

6. Cholestyramine possibly binding bacterial toxins improves symptoms.

Arguments for shared epithelial antigens ('autoimmunity')

1. Strong female predisposition (for collagenous colitis).

2. Frequent association with other autoimmune diseases and inflammatory arthropathies.

3. HLA patterns in lymphocytic colitis.

4. Therapeutic responses to anti-inflammatory and immunosuppressive agents.

5. Associations with IBD recently described.

Histopathogenesis and pathophysiology

Collagenous and lymphocytic colitis cause a secretory diarrhoea. The colonocytes cause a net fluid secretion due to an increase in the active chloride secretion, followed by a passive Na^+ transport; therefore the diarrhoea is not better during fasting. The composition of the collagen band has been studied in detail. The results suggest that the band is caused by a decreased degradation of type VI collagen.

This seems to be a very localized and rather aspecific phenomenon and may be caused by the diarrhoea itself as there seems to be no relation between the thickness of the band and the symptomatology. In contrast the inflammatory infiltrate in the lamina propria (mainly $CD4^+$ T cells) and the number of intraepithelial lymphocytes ($CD8^+$ T cells) suggest immune activation and correlate with disease activity.

What are the risk factors of developing the disease?

Risk factors and drugs potentially causing the disease

Non-steroidal anti-inflammatory agents (NSAIDs) have been mentioned as a possible cause. A clear causal relationship has been shown with a variety of other drugs (see Table 2). Our own recent study shows a statistically significant difference in smoking behaviour for the two conditions. Collagenous colitis patients are more likely to be active smokers while lymphocytic colitis patients are more often former smokers. These data are intriguing considering the opposite effects of nicotine use in Crohn's disease and ulcerative colitis, but need further confirmation. Early studies have suggested that heavy coffee drinkers were risk groups, but this has not been confirmed.

Table 2 Drugs causing collagenous colitis or lymphocytic colitis

RIEN	Collagenous	Lymphocytic
Ticlopidine	+	+++
Flutamide	−	++
Lansoprazole	+	++
Ranitidine	−	+
Cyclo 3 forte	+	+
Herbal preparations	+	−
NSAIDs	+	(+)

WHAT IS THE NATURAL HISTORY OF THESE CONDITIONS?

Prognosis and natural history

In contrast to earlier reports the prognosis of collagenous colitis and lymphocytic colitis is quite good. Irrespective of initial histology, spontaneous remission is frequent. Although fluctuations in the symptoms can occur, a relapse of symptoms after a period of remission is rare.

In a comparative study of both entities we found that, after a mean follow-up of 6 months, 59% of lymphocytic colitis patients compared to 34% of collagenous colitis patients reported a resolution of symptoms. Only 15% of lymphocytic and 26% of collagenous colitis patients had persistent important symptoms.

Longer-term follow-up figures are even better, with a remission rate of 25 out of 27 lymphocytic colitis patients after a median of 37.8 months and 14 out of 17 collagenous colitis patients in remission 47 months after diagnosis.

Histological remission rates are lower, especially for collagenous colitis. In lymphocytic colitis the histology returns to normal in 80% of patients in the long term. Good prospective histological data on collagenous colitis are lacking.

Bohr et al. reported five patients going into remission when becoming pregnant. This response can be due to a shift from Th1 to Th2 lymphocytes and cytokines similar to what has been observed and postulated in Crohn's disease.

About 20% of both collagenous colitis (CC) and lymphocytic colitis (LC) patients suffer from associated autoimmune conditions. No other significant co-morbidity or mortality is reported for both conditions. One study looked at the cancer risk in both entities. No cases of colorectal cancer were documented after 7 and 5 years follow-up in CC and LC respectively. In contrast, an increased relative risk for lung cancer in women with CC was noted, and an overall increased risk of malignancies in men with LC. These data should be confirmed however, and controlled for the potential role of smoking.

Recently a relationship with IBD was described. Out of a large pathological computer database at Mayo Clinic, 12 patients with IBD and microscopic colitis were found; 10 had CC and 2 LC. The diagnosis of IBD can precede, follow or coincide with CC or LC. Disease location of the IBD is colonic and usually pancolitis.

SHOULD WE TREAT ALL PATIENTS WITH COLLAGENOUS AND LYMPHOCYTIC COLITIS? WHAT IS THE APPROACH TO REFRACTORY CASES?

Treatment options and results

Take a detailed history for medication and herbal preparation use. Discontinue possible putative drugs (see Table 2).

Instruct the patient regarding the benign nature of the condition and relatively good prognosis. Consider dietary measures and non-specific antidiarrhoeal agents (loperamide, cholestyramine). If symptoms are not debilitating effective treatment options are available.

Budesonide should be considered standard treatment if persistent symptoms cause considerable discomfort.

Conventional steroid therapy will often induce a remission but symptoms are likely to recur when tapering. Budesonide is the most promising preparation, and appears to be effective even in steroid-refractory cases.

To date three randomized placebo-controlled trials, in total including 99 patients, are published that examined the role of budesonide in collagenous colitis. Overall they show a clinical response in 72–100% of patients treated with budesonide 9 mg for 6–8 weeks compared to 12–25% response in placebo-treated patients. Histological response is variable but a decrease of the subepithelial collagen layer and a decrease of the lymphoplasmocytic infiltrate in the lamina propria is observed in 46–69% of patients. In general patients responded within 2 weeks with no major side-effects; however, relapse is observed in 63–80% of patients when budesonide was stopped. Longer-term studies are not available. When budesonide cannot be tapered the use of azathioprine is reported as a steroid-sparing agent, as is common practice in other conditions such as IBD.

In lymphocytic colitis placebo-controlled studies are not available on the use of budesonide or on any other agent. In our personal experience with open-label use in 11 patients, 6 mg of budesonide was effective in 10/11 patients (91%) after a mean of 2.6 weeks (2–6 weeks). Budesonide was discontinued after 3–7 weeks of therapy. Only one of the 10 responders experienced a clinical relapse requiring extension of the budesonide therapy.

One open-label study reports beneficial effects of bismuth subsalicylate in a sufficient dose (600–800 mg/day) in a small group of patients. However, symptoms tend to reappear upon tapering of this drug. Safety concerns limit its long-term use; moreover bismuth is no longer commercially available in several countries.

A few case reports have been published concerning the beneficial effect of verapamil in collagenous colitis.

More aggressive immunosuppressive drugs (e.g. azathioprine and methotrexate) have occasionally been used, but are usually not indicated. One study mentions the use of azathioprine in steroid-dependent patients (see above).

Surgery with either diversion of the colon or colectomy should be considered only in very rare cases with life-threatening symptoms, but has been reported.

Table 3   Drugs with reported beneficial effects in collagenous and lymphocytic colitis

Steroids	*Motility agents*
Prednisolone	Loperamide
Budesonide	Somatostatin
Salicylates	
Sulphasalazine	*Miscellaneous*
Mesalazine (5-ASA)	Cholestyramine
Olsalazine	Mepacrine
	Bismuth subcitrate
Antibiotics	Verapamil
Metronidazole	Methotrexate
Erythromycin	Azathioprine
Penicillin	

MAIN CONCLUSIONS

1. Patients with unexplained chronic watery diarrhoea should undergo a colonoscopy with random biopsies to look for signs of collagenous colitis or lymphocytic colitis.

2. Main histological criteria are a dense mixed lymphoplasmocytic infiltrate in the lamina propria with a typical prominent subepithelial collagen band (measuring >10 μm) for collagenous colitis and an increased number of intraepithelial lymphocytes (>20 per 100 epithelial cells) for lymphocytic colitis.

3. Causes are unknown, but the histological abnormalities reflect an aspecific mild inflammatory reaction to a luminal antigen (often unknown, drugs, etc.) in a predisposed individual (autoimmune?).

4. The natural history is better for lymphocytic colitis than collagenous colitis. After about 6 months, 60% of lymphocytic and 34% of collagenous colitis patients are symptom-free. In the long term (after 3–4 years) almost all patients do well.

5. Budesonide has become the standard of care with three placebo-controlled randomized trials showing efficacy. In collagenous colitis 9 mg for 6–8 weeks is effective short term in most patients, but relapse occurs frequently after stopping. In lymphocytic colitis controlled evidence is lacking but personal open-label experience with lower dose and shorter duration of therapy is excellent. Longer-term data are awaited.

Bibliography

Agnarsdottir M, Gunnlaugsson O, Orvar KB et al. Collagenous and lymphocytic colitis in Iceland. Dig Dis Sci. 2002;47:1122–8.

Aigner T, Neureiter D, Müller S, Küspert G, Belke J, Kirchner T. Extracellular matrix composition and gene expression in collagenous colitis. Gastroenterology. 1997;113:136–43.

Armes J, Gee DC, Macrae FA, Schroeder W, Bhathal PS. Collagenous colitis: jejunal and colorectal pathology. J Clin Pathol. 1992;45:784–7.

Baert F, Schmit A, D'Haens G et al. Budesonide in collagenous colitis: a prospective double-blind placebo-controlled trial with histological follow-up. Gastroenterology. 2002;122:20–5.

Baert F, Wouters K, D'haens G et al. Lymphocytic colitis: a distinct clinical entity? A clinicopathological confrontation of lymphocytic and collagenous colitis. Gut. 1999;45:375–81.

Baugerie L, Lubonski J, Brousse N et al. Drug induced lymphocytic colitis. Gut. 1994;35:426–8.

Baugerie L, Patey N, Brousse N. Ranitidine, diarrhoea and lymphocytic colitis. Gut. 1995;37:708–11.

Bayless TM, Giardiello FM, Lazenby A, Yardley JH. Collagenous colitis. Mayo Clin Proc. 1987;62:665–71.

Berrebi D, Sauter A, Flejou JF et al. Ticlodipine induced colitis: a histological study including apoptosis. J Clin Pathol. 1998;51:280–3.

Bogomoletz WV. Collagenous, microscopic, and lymphocytic colitis. An evolving concept. Virchows Arch. 1994;424:573–9.

Bohr J, Olesen M, Tysk C et al. Collagenous and lymphocytic colitis: a clinical and histopathological review. Can J Gastroenterol. 2000;14:943–7.

Bohr J, Olesen M, Tysk C, Jämerot G. Budesonide and bismuth in microscopic colitis. Gut. 1999;45:A202.

Bohr J, Tysk C, Eriksson S, Abrahamsson H, Järnerot G. Collagenous colitis: a retrospective study of clinical presentation and treatment in 163 patients. Gut. 1996;39:846–51.

Bohr J, Tysk C, Eriksson S et al. Collagenous colitis in Örebro, Sweden: an epidemiological study 1984–1993. Gut. 1995;37:394–7.

Bohr J, Tysk C, Yang P, Danielsson D, Järnerot G. Autoantibodies and immunoglobulins in collagenous colitis. Gut. 1996;39:73–6.

Bonderup OK, Hansen JB, Birket-Schmit L, Vestergaard V, Tegibaerg PS, Fallingborg J. Budesonide treatment of collagenous colitis: a randomized, double-blind placebo-controlled trial. Gut. 2001;49:A1906.

Bowling TE, Price AB, Al-Adnani M, Fairclough PD, Menzies-Gow N, Silk DBA. Interchange between collagenous and lymphocytic colitis in severe disease with auto-immune associations requiring colectomy: a case-report. Gut. 1996;38:788–91.

Campieri M, Ferguson A, Doe W, Persson T, Nilsson LG. Oral budesonide is as effective as oral prednisolone in active Crohn's disease. Gut. 1197;41:209–14.

Carpentier HA, Tremaine WJ, Batts KP, Czaja AJ. Sequential histologic evaluations in collagenous colitis. Correlations with disease behavior and sampling strategy. Dig Dis Sci. 1992;37:1903–9.

Chan JL, Tersmette AC, Offerhaus GJA, Gruber SB, Giardello FM. Cancer risk in patients with lymphocytic and collagenous colitis. Gastroenterology. 1998;114:G1462.

Dafnis G, Blomqvist P, Påhlman L et al. The introduction and development of colonoscopy within a defined population in Sweden. Scand J Gastroenterol. 2000;35:765–71.

Delarive J, Saraga E, Dorta G, Blum AL. Budesonide in the treatment of collagenous colitis. Digestion. 1998;59:364–6.

Edsbäcker S, Lundin P, Larsson P, Wollmer P. Targeted delivery of oral budesonide (Entocort capsules) in healthy volunteers and Crohn's disease patients (abstr.). Bangkok: World Congress of Gastroenterology, 2002.

Ekbom A, Helmick C, Zack M et al. The epidemiology of inflammatory bowel disease: a large, population-based study in Sweden. Gastroenterology. 1991;100:350–8.

Fernandez-Banares F, Salas A, Forne M et al. Incidence of collagenous and lymphocytic colitis: a 5-year population-based study. Am J Gastroenterol. 1999;94:418–23.

Fine K, Ogunji F, Lee E, Lafon G, Tanzi M. Randomized, double-blind placebo-controlled trial of bismuth subsalicylate for microscopic colitis (abstr). Gastroenterology. 1999;116:A880.

Gardiello FM, Lazenby AJ, Bayless TM et al. Lymphocytic (microscopic) colitis: clinicopathological study of 18 patients and comparison to collagenous colitis. Dig Dis Sci. 1989;34:1730–8.

Gardiello FM, Lazenby AJ. The atypical colitides. Gastroenterol Clin N Am. 1999;28:479–90.

Giardiello FM, Lazenby AJ, Yardley JH et al. Increased HLA A1 and diminished HLA A3 in lymphocytic colitis compared to controls and in patients with collagenous colitis. Dig Dis Sci. 1992;37:496–9.

Greenberg GR, Feagan BG, Martin F et al. Oral budesonide for active Crohn's disease. N Engl J Med. 1194;331:836–41.

Günther U, Schuppan D, Bauer M et al. Fibrogenesis and fibrolysis in collagenous colitis: patterns of procollagen types I and IV, matrix-metalloproteinase-1 and 13, and TIMP-1gene expression. Am J Pathol. 1999;155:493–503.

Järnerot G, Tysk C, Bohr J, Eriksson S. Collagenous colitis and faecal stream diversion. Gastroenterology. 1995;109:449–55.

Jessurun J, Yardley JH, Giardello FM, Hamilton SR, Bayless T. Chronic colitis with thickening of the subepithelial collagen layer (collagenous colitis): histopathological findings in 15 patients. Hum Pathol. 1987;18:839–48.

Lanyi B, Dries V, Dienes HP, Kruis W. Therapy for prednisone refractory collagenous colitis with budesonide. Int J Colorectal Dis. 1999;14:58–61.

Lapidus A, Bernell O, Hellers G et al. Incidence of Crohn's disease in Stockholm County 1955–1989. Gut. 1997;41:480–6.

Lazenby AJ, Yardley JH, Giardiello FM, Jessurun J, Bayless TM. Lymphocytic colitis ("microscopic") colitis: a comparative histopathologic study with particular reference to collagenous colitis. Hum Pathol. 1989;20:18–28.

Lee E, Schiller LR, Vendrell D, Santa-Ana CA, Fordtran JS. Subepithelial collagen thickness in colon specimens from patients with microscopic colitis and collagenous colitis. Gastroenterology. 1992;103:1790–6.

Lindberg E, Järnerot G. The incidence of Crohn's disease is not decreasing in Sweden. Scand J Gastroenterol. 1991;26:495–500.

Lindström CG. Collagenous colitis with watery diarrhoea: a new entity? Pathol Eur. 1976;11:87–9.

Mäkinen M, Niemelä S, Lethola J, Karrtunen TJ. Collagenous colitis and *Yersinia enterocolitica* infection. Dig Dis Sci. 1998;43:1341–6.

Marsh MN. Gluten, major histocompatibility complex, and the small intestine. A molecular and immunobiologic approach to the spectrum of gluten sensitivity ("celiac sprue"). Gastroenterology. 1992;102:330–54.

Martinez Aviles P, Gisbert Moya C, Berbegal Serra J et al. Ticlopidine induced lymphocytic colitis (letter). Med Clin Barc. 1996;106:317.

Meier PN, Otto P, Ritter M, Stolte M. Collagenous duodenitis and ileitis in a patient with collagenous colitis. Leber Magen Darm. 1991;21:231–2.

Mosnier JF, Larvol L, Barge J et al. Lymphocytic and collagenous colitis: an immunohistochemical study. Am J Gastroenterol. 1996;91:709–13.

Mullhaupt B, Güller U, Anabitarte M et al. Lymphocytic colitis: clinical presentation and long term course. Gut. 1998;43:629–33.

Raclot G, Queneau PE, Ottignon Y et al. Incidence of collagenous colitis. A retrospective study in the east of France. Gastroenterology. 1994;106:A23.

Riddel RH, Tanaka M, Mazzoleni G. Non-steroidal anti-inflammatory drugs as a possible cause of collagenous colitis: a case control study. Gut. 1992;33:683–6.

Rutgeerts P, Löfberg R, Malchow H et al. A comparison of budesonide with prednisolone from active Crohn's disease. N Engl J Med. 1994;331:842–5.

Schmeck-Lindenau HJ, Kürtz W, Heine M. Lymphocytic colitis during ticlodipine therapy (letter). Dtsch Med Wochenschr. 1998;123:479.

Sloth H, Bisgaard C, Grove A. Collagenous colitis: a prospective trial of prednisolone in six patients. J Intern Med. 1991;229:443–6.

Snook J. Are the inflammatory bowel diseases autoimmune disorders? Gut. 1990;31:961–3.

Stahle-Bäckdhl M, Malm J, Veress B, Benoni C, Bruce K, Egesten A. Increased presence of eosinophilic granulocytes expressing transforming growth factor-β1 in collagenous colitis. Scand J Gastroenterol. 2000;35:742–6.

Stolte M, Ritter M, Borchard F, Koch-Scherrer G. Collagenous gastroduodenitis and collagenous colitis. Encoscopy. 1990;22:186–7.

Sylwestrowicz T, Kelly JK, Hwang WS, Shaffer EA. Collagenous and microscopic colitis: the watery diarrhea-colitis syndrome. Am J Gastroenterol. 1989;84:763–8.

Taha Y, Kraaz W, Lööf L. Förekomst av kollagen kolt i biopsier vid koloskopi med makroskopiskt normal slemhinna (Swedish). Sv Läkaresällskapets handl Hygiea. 1995;104:A167.

Tanaka M, Mazzaloni G, Riddell RH. Distribution of collagenous colitis: utility of flexible sigmoidoscopy. Gut. 1992;33:65–70.

Thomson A. Microscopic colitis – no longer an appropriate term? Am J Gastroenterol. 1998;93: 524–6.

Thomson O, Cortot A, Jewell D et al. A comparison of budesonide and mesalamine for active Crohn's disease. N Engl J Med. 1998;339:370–4.

Tromm A, Griga T, Möllmann HW, May B, Müller KM, Fisseler-Eckhoff A. Budesonide for the treatment of collagenous colitis: first results of a pilot trial. Am J Gastroenterol. 1999;94: 1871–5.

Tysk C, Järnerot G. Ulcerative proctocolitis in Örebro, Sweden. A retrospective epidemiology study, 1963–1987. Scand J Gastroenterol. 1992;27:945–50.

Ung KA, Gillberg R, Kilander A, Abrahamsson H. Role of bile acids and bile acid binding agents in patients with collagenous colitis. Gut. 2000;46:170–5.

Veress B, Lofberg R, Bergman L, Microscopic colitis syndrome. Gut. 1195;36:880–6.

Zins B, Sandborn W, Tremaine W. Collagneous colitis and lymphocytic colitis: subject review and therapeutic alternatives. Am J Gastroenterol. 1995;90:1394–400.

7
Budesonide in refractory sprue

S. DAUM and J.-D. SCHULZKE

INTRODUCTION

Refractory sprue (RS) is a heterogeneous group of diseases and is defined by persisting villous atrophy and usually an increase of intra-epithelial lymphocytes in the small bowel in spite of a strict gluten-free diet (GFD)[1,2] Some of these diseases can be treated by specific therapies such as antibiotics in tropical sprue, immunoglobulin substitution in common variable immunodeficiency or acid suppression in hypergastrinaemia. However, in the remaining group of patients suffering from RS, therapeutic strategies are not well defined[2]. Among these are patients with autoimmune enteropathy and RS with or without signs of an early EATCL, e.g. loss of antigens or clonality of the T-cell receptor gene[3-5]. Immunosuppressive therapy has proven to be successful in some of these cases and in a recent prospective report[6]. In other reports immunosuppressive therapy was less convincing[7,8]. One reason might be the presence of a clonal T-cell population that proliferates under immunosuppression. Steroid treatment has mostly been effective even in patients with underlying early EATCL[4]. However, this therapy is handicapped by long-term side-effects of high systemic steroid doses which may be overcome using budesonide. The present study aimed to evaluate the effect of budesonide, a locally acting steroid, in patients with RS, which has not been investigated so far. Thus, the clinical benefit of treatment with budesonide was investigated retrospectively in a small group of patients with RS.

METHODS

Patients

Six patients with RS and one patient with autoimmune enteropathy, who were refractory more than 1 year to a strict GFD, were included (Table 2). Other reasons for persisting villous atrophy were excluded (cf. Table 1). Six of seven patients started on prednisolone per os and were changed to 9–12 mg budesonide per day. One patient was directly started on 9 mg budesonide per day. General status, weight, frequency of bowel movements and stool were analysed.

Table 1 Other reasons for refractory villous atrophy and clinical tests

Blind loop syndrome	Glucose H_2-breath test
CVID	Serum antibodies (IgG, IgA, IgM)
Hypergastrinaemia	Serum gastrin
Giardiasis	Stool tests for *Giardia lamblia*
Collagenous sprue	Histology (tenascin staining)
Tropical sprue	Antibiotics and folic acid in travellers
Cow milk, egg and soya intolerance	Exclusion diet
Autoimmune enteropathy	Enterocyte antibodies

Histology

Biopsies were taken from the duodenum during upper gastrointestinal endoscopy and were fixed in 4% formalin and embedded in paraffin for morphological analysis. Serial sections (3 µm) were stained with haematoxylin and eosin (HE) or dewaxed for immunostaining. The number or intraepithelial lymphocytes (IELs) per 100 epithelial cells was counted in duodenal biopsies (in HE as well as in CD3 immunostained sections).

Immunohistochemistry

Sections of formalin-fixed, paraffin-embedded tissue were used for immunohistochemistry applying the immunoalkaline phosphatase (APAAP) method using the following antibodies: βF1 (TCR β-chain) from T-cell Sciences (Cambridge, USA), 123C3 (CD56) from Monosan (Uden, Netherlands), and 1F6 (CD4), C8-144 (CD8) and CD3 (polyclonal) all from DAKO (Glostrup, Denmark). Pretreatment was done using high-pressure cooking for antigen retrieval in a 10 mmol/L citrate buffer, pH 6.0.

Clonality analysis of T-cell receptor-γ (TCR-γ) in IEL in refractory sprue (RF)

A semi-nested polymerase chain reaction (PCR) was performed for the detection of clonal TCR-γ gene rearrangements. In the first round of amplification two separate reactions were carried out employing the same Vg1-8 consensus primer in conjunction with the Jg primer JGT1/2 and JGT3, respectively[5].

Clinical response to budesonide

Positive response was documented in case of stable clinical status after changing from prednisolone to budesonide or in case of further improvement. Antigenic loss of IELs was assumed when more than 50% of IELs were negative for CD8 or TCR-β.

Table 2 Refractory sprue (RS) type I and type II

Patient	Gender	Age (years)	Diagnosis	CD-Ab	IEL	Initial response to GFD	TCR-γ clonality	Antigen (CD8, TCR-β)	Budesonide response
S.R.	Female	18	Autoimmune enteropathy	Negative	15	No	Polyclonal	Present	Yes
R.K.	Male	61	Refractory sprue I	Negative	50	No	Polyclonal	Present	Yes
R.D.	Male	43	Refractory sprue I	Positive	63	+	Polyclonal	Present	Yes
E.K.	Male	64	Refractory sprue I	Positive	70	+	Polyclonal	Present	Yes
H.V.	Male	61	Sprue-like TCL	Positive	87	+	Monoclonal	Loss	Yes
M.R.	Female	47	CD4+ TCL	Positive	20	No	Monoclonal	(CD4)	Yes
H.H.	Male	57	Sprue-like TCL, later EATCL	Positive	120	+	Monoclonal	Loss	No

RESULTS

The data of the seven patients included, and the outcome, are shown in Table 2. The first patient with autoimmune hepatitis was initially assumed to suffer from coeliac disease, but did not respond to 12 months GFD. As she had negative serum sprue antibodies (tTG IgA), a second round of investigations was started revealing anti-enterocyte antibody titres as well as a type I autoimmune hepatitis (ANA-positive). The duodenal histology showed a normal IEL count and a complete loss of goblet cells in the flat small intestinal mucosa (total villous atrophy). After changing the diagnosis to autoimmune enteropathy the GFD was stopped and 40 mg prednisolone per day was started orally. This led to a cessation of the diarrhoea (from 10 stools per day to two stools per day) and the patient started to gain body weight again (the initial body weight loss amounted to 17 kg). Subsequently, the steroid therapy was switched to 9 mg budesonide per day, and this led to a further increase in body weight; then azathioprine was started.

Three of the six RS patients had a polyclonal TCR-γ gene repertoire of their increased IEL and showed no loss of antigen in immune histochemistry (i.e. more than 50% were CD8-positive). These three patients with RS type I all responded to budesonide. One was switched to azathioprine but had to be withdrawn due to azathioprine-induced pancreatitis. The other two are still on budesonide 9 mg per day, but it is planned to start azathioprine.

Patients 5 to 7 in Table 2 suffer from RS type II. Patient 5 presented with diarrhoea and a 2 kg loss in body weight. His sprue antibody test was positive and he initially responded to a GFD clinically and histologically. Subsequently, his clinical status worsened again in spite of the strict diet; then he was re-evaluated and it was found that he had a monoclonal TCR-γ gene repertoire as well as antigen loss; therefore, prednisolone was started. In an oral dose of 40 mg per day, prednisolone improved his clinical performance and he started to gain weight again. The switch to 9 mg budesonide was successful and he has been stable on this budesonide dose for 2 years.

Patient 6 presented with diarrhoea, total villous atrophy and a negative serum sprue–antibody test. She was *a priori* refractory to a GFD but had a rare histological appearance with only 20 IEL per 100 enterocytes which were CD8-negative but stained for CD4. Therefore, clonality analysis was performed, revealing monoclonality of the TCR-γ gene. Budesonide was then given (9 mg per day orally), which improved her clinical performance and her mucosal architecture. So far no further medication is considered, since the patient is doing well on this medication.

Patient 7 also presented with severe diarrhoea and a pronouced loss in body weight. His sprue–antibody test was positive. His total villous atrophy, however, did not respond to a GFD. The subsequent analysis of his IEL revealed both antigen loss as well as monoclonality of the TCR-γ gene. Steroids did not improve his villous architecture or diarrhoea; also, a CD25 antibody therapy was not successful. He is now planned to receive chemotherapy (CHOP).

DISCUSSION

Our present study reports for the first time successful treatment of patients with refractory sprue (RS) type I and type II with the topical steroid budesonide.

In our definition RS I and RS II are two distinct groups of patients among the large and heterogeneous group of patients not responding to a GFD when diagnosed with villous atrophy[1,2]. As refractory sprue is also often used for all patients with villous atrophy who had not responded to a GFD, we will define this in more detail. First, one has to ensure that the GFD is strictly adhered to, and that there was enough time for the recovery. Some patients need up to 2 years to recover, even if most re-evaluations in the clinical routine are made as early as 12 months. Secondly, we have to rule out other reasons for a GFD-refractory villous atrophy. A list of such other reasons is summarized in Table 1. While some of these are easy to address, e.g. common variable immunodeficiency by testing serum antibody class concentrations, hypergastrinaemia by measuring serum gastrin levels or the blind loop syndrome by performing the H_2-breath test with D-glucose, others are much more difficult to detect, e.g. autoimmune enteropathy or food allergies. In this case indirect evidence for an originally coeliac sprue-derived refractory sprue may be useful; this can be: (a) a previous course of gluten-sensitive sprue (secondary refractory sprue); (b) positive serum sprue antibodies, or (c) a positive test for HLA-DQ2 (which is found in 90% of coeliac patients but only in 20% of the normal population[9]. If one cannot obtain further evidence for a coeliac-derived refractory atrophy in this manner, it is justified to test patients for food allergy including an exclusion dietary programme and to test for anti-enterocyte antibodies. As far as the latter is concerned, one should bear in mind that the sensitivity of this antibody test is far from 100% in adults. The coincidence with other autoimmune disease may help in this respect.

To follow such a diagnostic algorithm is the best we can do today, to identify patients with a coeliac disease-derived diet-refractory status which can then be subsequently subdivided into two groups, RS type I and type II. This is achieved by analysing the clonality of the TCR-γ gene and antigens such as CD8 in IELs which are lost during transformation of these cells towards a coeliac-associated intestinal T-cell lymphoma (EATCL). Thus, in contrast to type I RS, type II RS represents an early T-cell lymphoma, the cell clone of which is in this stage only diffusely spread over the small intestine, and still has no condensed manifestion in the form of an overt T-cell lymphoma. Although we have only one prospective study, and no long-term observations on this topic, there seems to be little tendency of RS type I patients to proceed to the type II status in the first 2–3 years of follow-up. Therefore, it seems justified to evaluate the therapeutic benefit of medications in the future separately in type I and type II RS.

As the main result of our present retrospective analysis, the topical steroid budesonide in the Entocort® formula was effective in stardard doses in most type I- and type II-refractory sprue patients. All three type I and two of three type II RS patients responded to budesonide.

The subsequent therapy concept, however, is different between the two groups. Although Maurino et al.[6] presented data on the clinical benefit of type I and II RS patients on azathioprine, immunosuppressive therapy for patients with a premalignant condition (RS II) should await further prospective and long-term data. In type I RS, topical steroids may be used to reduce systemic steroid side-effects and to cover the time until the immunosuppressive therapy has reached its final efficacy, which in the case of azathioprine can need many months[6]. Then, budesonide, as with prednisolone in the past, should be slowly reduced and finally withdrawn. However, it may be possible that busesonide could represent a long-term reserve medication in RS type I patients who finally do not remain stable on the immunosuppressive monotherapy. In type II RS patients we prefer a stepwise escalating therapy strategy, and keep our patients as long on budesonide as they continue to respond clinically. Thus, we finally start chemotherapy (CHOP) only in those who do not respond to steroids in RS II. However, other groups treat type II RS patients early with chemotherapy, and there is to date no final decision on this question, since prospective data are lacking.

Thus, taken together, our retrospective study on a small group of refractory sprue patients is the first report on a successful topical steroid therapy in this group of patients. The promising result, with six of seven patients responding, seems to indicate that budesonide (Entocort®) is a useful alternative for prednisolone to reduce systemic steroid side-effects in both type I and type II refractory sprue. However, prospective studies with significant numbers of patients are necessary in this field before final conclusions can be drawn. So far we would propose budesonide: (a) for patients with RS type I, in order to reduce systemic steroid therapy before or while starting azathioprine; (b) for patients with RS type I, who cannot receive immunosuppressive therapy, and (c) for patients with RS type II (sprue-like intestinal T-cell lymphoma), who are not suitable for chemotherapy or have clinically stabilized.

References

1. Mulder C, Wahab P, Moshaver B et al. Refractory coeliac disease: a window between coeliac disease and enteropathy associated T-cell lymphoma. Scand J Gastroenterol. 2000;35:32–7.
2. Ryan B, Kelleher D. Refractory celiac disease. Gastroenterology. 2000;119:243–51.
3. Carbonnel F, Grollet-Bioul L, Brouet J et al. Are complicated forms of celiac disease cryptic T-cell lymphomas? Blood. 1998;92:3879–86.
4. Cellier C, Delabesse E, Helmer C et al. Refractory sprue, coeliac disease, and enteropathy-associated T-cell lymphoma. Lancet. 2000;356:203–8.
5. Daum S, Weiss D, Hummel M et al. Frequency of clonal intraepithelial T-lymphocyte proliferations in enteropathy-type intestinal T-cell lymphoma, celiac disease and refractory sprue. Gut. 2001;49:804-12.
6. Maurino E, Niveloni S, Chernavsky A et al. Azathioprine in refractory sprue: results from a prospective open-label study. Am J Gastroenterol. 2002;97:2595–602.
7. Wahab P, Crusius J, Meijer J et al. Cyclosporine in the treatment of adults with refractory coeliac disease – an open pilot study. Aliment Pharmacol Ther. 2000;14:767–74.
8. Mulder C, Wahab P, Meijer J et al. A pilot study of recombinant human interleukin-10 in adults with refractory coeliac disease. Eur J Gastroenterol Hepatol. 2001;13:1183–8.
9. Wahnschaffe U, Ullrich R, Riecken E-O et al. Celiac disease-like antibodies in a subgroup of patients with irritable bowel syndrome. Gastroenterology. 2001;121:1329–38.

8
Potential use of budesonide in food hypersensitivity

M. RAITHEL, M. WEIDENHILLER, V. WILKEN, J. HOCHBERGER, S. T. MUEHLDORFER and E. G. HAHN

INTRODUCTION

Infiltrates of mast cells with signs of activation and degranulation have been observed in lesions of both inflammatory bowel disease (IBD) and gastrointestinally mediated allergy (GMA)[1-5]. By secretion of a great plethora of different types of mediators, e.g. preformed mediators such as histamine and serotonin, newly generated mediators (arachidonic acid metabolites), as well as proteases and cytokines, mast cells of the gut may exert some pathophysiological effects in chronic and allergic intestinal inflammation. While the stimuli (nutritive antigens) and the pathogenic role of intestinal mast cell populations (mucosal type and connective tissue type) are well established in allergic enteropathy, the pathophysiological triggers for mast cell degranulation in ulcerative colitis (UC) and Crohn's disease are not yet fully known[4-6].

Since intestinal mast cells have the potential to aggravate or induce gut mucosal inflammation (mast cell leucocyte cascade[6]), to interact with B cells and eosinophils, the effect of budesonide, a topically effective steroid, was studied in a group of patients with UC and GMA in terms of mediator secretion from intestinal mast cells and eosinophils.

Although the topical steroid budesonide is well known to exhibit strong inhibitory effects on eosinophils in the bronchial mucosa of asthmatics, which intimately interact with mast cell subtypes[6-8], the effect of budesonide on living human gut mucosal tissue has not yet been studied. This study was therefore constructed to detect the secretion of a highly mast cell-associated protease, tryptase (T) and an eosinophilic specific protein, eosinophilic cationic protein (ECP) from viable gut mucosal samples in the presence or absence of budesonide. This project should provide first experimental hints as to the use of budesonide in conditions other than IBD, e.g. food hypersensitivity or other various disease types with predominant mast cell or eosinophil activity.

MATERIAL AND METHODS

Patient groups

The study included 176 biopsies of 12 untreated patients with UC and 22 untreated patients with GMA. Age (mean $\pm$ SD), sex and the number of patients (biopsies) investigated for each group are shown in Table 1. The study protocol was approved by the local ethics committee (No. 331) and all patients gave their informed consent to participate.

The diagnosis of UC in 12 patients was established by clinical, radiological, endoscopic and histological criteria. Stool cultures were shown to be negative in all patients. Patients underwent colonoscopy for the actual assessment of activity and extension of disease or for surveillance colonoscopy. Four or five mucosal samples were taken from terminal ileum and/or ascending colon for measurement of T and ECP release in the culture medium, either in the presence or absence of budesonide.

Twenty-two patients with confirmed GMA (double-blind, placebo-controlled food challenge, DBPCFC) also took part in the study. All 22 allergy patients (100%) presented with postprandial abdominal discomfort (diarrhoea or loose stools, pain, vomiting), while extraintestinal atopic symptoms such as allergic rhinoconjunctivitis, skin reactions and asthma bronchiale occurred at a lower frequency (nine of 22 patients, 40.9%). Sensitization(s) to food antigens were found either by skin prick tests (27%), by demonstration of food-specific IgE antibodies in serum (43%) or in gastrointestinal lavage fluid (41%)[9]. DBPCFC was performed using a nasogastric tube, and freshly prepared foodstuffs were administered three times daily to the patient[9]. Oral provocation was monitored and assessed by evaluation of all subjective and objective symptoms as well as by continuous measurement of allergy mediators in serum and urine[9]. A significant clinical reaction was defined as a mean symptom score above six points and/or an increase of allergy mediators more than 40% compared to the previous test day without symptoms[9-11].

At the time of colonoscopy no patient had been under antiallergic, immunosuppressive or steroid treatment for 2 weeks at least. Patients were prepared for colonoscopy using a commercial polyethyleneglycol solution. To facilitate colonoscopy, benzodiazepines (midazolam, diazepam) and meperidine were used at a dose of 2.5–10 mg (midazolam, diazepam) and 25–150 mg (meperidine), respectively in 14/22 patients (64%) with food allergy and in 8/12 patients (67%) with UC[4].

Table 1 Patients' characteristics for analysis of mast cell and eosinophil mediator secretion with or without budesonide from living gut mucosal samples

Patient group	Age; male/female	Biopsies
Gastrointestinally mediated allergy (GMA) ($n = 22$)	37 ± 12; 10/12	114 samples
Ulcerative colitis (UC) ($n = 12$)	34 ± 8; 8/4	62 samples

MUCOSA OXYGENATION OF COLORECTAL SAMPLES: T AND ECP RELEASE IN THE PRESENCE OR ABSENCE OF BUDESONIDE

In addition to biopsy samples for routine histology a total of 176 mucosal biopsies (four or five samples/patient) were taken endoscopically from the terminal ileum and/or the ascending colon for measurement of mediator secretion[4,5]. Terminal ileum and ascending colon were chosen for this study as they had previously been found to harbour the highest tissue content of eosinophil and mast cell mediators physiologically, to show the most dense infiltration rates of eosinophils and mast cells histologically and because budesonide is primarily released from its drug formulation in this regions.

To purify samples from mucus, faeces or foodstuffs biopsies were immediately placed (<10 s after endoscopic removal) into an oxygenated transport medium. They were separately placed into a Hanks solution (4 ml, pH 6, pO_2 85–90 mmHg) for 45 min. Since mucosal ischaemia causes a disturbed mediator response, biopsy incubation was continuously performed by mucosa oxygenation[4,5]. To avoid ischaemic conditions the Hanks solution, as well as the following culture medium, were bubbled with a steady flow of room air, ensuring a sufficient oxygen pressure inside the tissue of 85–90 mmHg as published previously[4,5].

After washing the samples within the transport medium, wet weights of biopsies were measured by the use of a microbalance (Sartorius, Göttingen, Germany) and then placed in the culture medium for measuring the spontaneous mediator release during 4 h of mucosa oxygenation[4,5]. The incubation medium contained 4 ml of a modified Hanks solution (supplemented with 25 mM Hepes buffer, 1% fetal calf serum and 0.3% human serum albumin). Temperature (37°C), oxygen pressure (pO_2 85–95 mmHg) and pH (6.9–7.0) were maintained stable by mucosa oxygenation throughout the whole incubation period of 4 h[4,5].

Part of the biopsies (two or three samples) from each patient was cultured with budesonide (1 mM, final concentration within the culture medium; Astra Wedel, Germany) and the other part (two or three samples) without budesonide served as control. At day 1 the budesonide was added to the samples at the beginning of the mucosa oxygenation, already in the transport medium (Hanks solution) before weighing of biopsies. After weighing the biopsies were placed in the oxygenated culture medium at time 0 min. T and ECP release were then followed for 4 h (first culture, Tables 2 and 3) in the presence or absence of budesonide[4,5].

Afterwards the biopsies were each taken in a new fresh oxygenated medium, which contained budesonide or not, corresponding to the first release period. Thus, samples were cultured overnight (20 h). T and ECP release were then again followed 24 h after endoscopic sample-taking, after having put the samples into a new fresh culture medium (as done at day 1). The mediator secretion was then followed again for 4 h at day 2 (second culture, Tables 2 and 3), again either in the presence or absence of budesonide.

During every culture period (first and second culture at day 1 and 2), each 400 µl of the supernatant were removed at time points 0, 30, 60, 120 and 240 min, respectively.

The released amounts of T or ECP were later calculated for the actual incubation volume by a GW-BASIC software program. Since mast cell mediators

Table 2 Spontaneous tryptase release from intact colorectal mucosa of patients with gastrointestinally mediated allergy (GMA) and ulcerative colitis (UC)*

	Spontaneous tryptase release	Anti-IgE induced- tryptase release
First culture: 1 h after sample taking		
GMA without budesonide	1.1 ± 0.2 (4.6%)	1.4 ± 0.3 (9.6%)
GMA with budesonide	0.9 ± 0.1 (2.9%)	0.8 ± 0.1 (3.0%)
Ulcerative colitis without budesonide	1.5 ± 0.4 (3.4%)	1.3 ± 0.2 (8.8%)
Ulcerative colitis with budesonide	1.1 ± 0.2 (3.3%)	2.1 ± 0.8 (3.7%)
Second culture: 24 h after sample taking		
GMA without budesonide	3.4 ± 0.6 (18.4%)	0.8 ± 0.1 (4.1%)
GMA with budesonide	3.0 ± 1.2 (10.6%)	0.9 ± 0.7 (2.6%)
Ulcerative colitis without budesonide	3.0 ± 0.5 (7.9%)	2.2 ± 0.5 (7.7%)
Ulcerative colitis with budesonide	2.0 ± 0.3 (8.6%)	2.3 ± 0.7 (5.0%)

*The rate of mediator release (mean ± SEM) is given both as absolute value (ng/mg wet weight) and as median percentage release (in parentheses) of the total tissue mediator content

Table 3 Spontaneous release of eosinophilic cationic protein from intact colorectal mucosa of patients with gastrointestinally mediated allergy (GMA) and ulcerative colitis (UC)*

	Spontaneous ECP release	Anti-IgE-induced- ECP release
First culture: 1 h after sample taking		
GMA without budesonide	3.5 ± 1.0 (18.8%)	8.0 ± 5.2 (20.8%)
GMA with budesonide	2.5 ± 1.0 (11.2%)	2.3 ± 0.5 (19.8%)
Ulcerative colitis without budesonide	5.4 ± 2.3 (13.0%)	3.3 ± 1.0 (11.9%
Ulcerative colitis with budesonide	3.7 ± 1.5 (10.7%)	5.1 ± 1.8 (10.7%)
Second culture: 24 h after sample taking		
GMA without budesonide	1.4 ± 0.3 (20.4%)	6.0 ± 2.5 (22.9%)
GMA with budesonide	2.0 ± 0.6 (15.6%)	1.5 ± 0.3 (16.1%)
Ulcerative colitis without budesonide	6.0 ± 3.8 (17.5%)	–
Ulcerative colitis with budesonide	4.2 ± 2.5 (14.2%)	–

*The rate of mediator release (mean ± SEM) is given both as absolute value (ng/mg wet weight) and as median percentage release (in parentheses) of the total tissue mediator content

can have negative feedback effects on mast cell activation, the incubation medium was corrected to a volume of 4 ml at the time point 60 min by addition of 1200 μl of incubation medium with or without budesonide. The aliquots of each time point were immediately collected on ice and centrifuged (7 min, +4°C, 400g). Thereafter supernatants were stored at –20°C until performance of the T or ECP fluoroenzyme immunoassay (Unicap System, Pharmacia, Freiburg, Germany). Intra-assay and inter-assay variation of T and ECP measurement were 6.1% (T) and 7.8% (ECP), or 13.1% (T) and 11.2% (ECP), respectively.

The effective increase of mediator secretion resulted from addition of the T or ECP amounts released during the complete incubation period. This reflects the net mediator secretion, which is given as nanograms mediator/milligram wet weight $\pm$ standard error of the mean (SEM).

Intra-individual variation of spontaneous T secretion from different samples taken from the lower gastrointestinal tract of colorectal mucosa from GMA amounted to $19\pm9\%$ and in UC to $26.2\pm12\%$, while ECP secretion was $11.2\pm3\%$ and $14.7\pm9\%$, respectively.

For descriptive statistics the mean $\pm$ SEM are given, while the mediator release as a percentage of the total tissue mediator content (from one biopsy) is shown in parentheses. Statistical comparisons were made by the U-test (Wilcoxon test); significance levels are given in parentheses.

RESULTS

Gastrointestinally mediated allergy

Release of mast cell T as parameter of mast cell function

The rates of spontaneous and anti-IgE-induced T release in GMA are given in Table 2. Although there were no statistically significant differences between T secretion without or with budesonide, T release in GMA was slightly inhibited when budesonide was present in the culture medium.

The increase of the net T secretion induced by the given anti-IgE dilution of 1/40 is small (as compared to the release values of intestinal eosinophils), but may also be seen with the percentage value of 9.6%. Interestingly, budesonide inhibited such a functional immunological T release, as both release parameters (net mediator secretion and percentage value) remain low in the first and second culture.

Release of ECP as parameter of eosinophil function

The rates of spontaneous and anti-IgE-induced ECP release in GMA are given in Table 3. In contrast to mast cells the given anti-IgE concentration induced a tremendous amount of ECP secretion within 4 h of cultivation, both in the first and second culture. While budesonide was able to slightly inhibit the spontaneous ECP secretion in the first culture at day 1, release values after 24 h at day 2 were similar.

The most impressive effect of budesonide, however, was its inhibitory effect on intestinal eosinophil function in the presence of anti-IgE. Budesonide clearly inhibited immunologically induced ECP secretion even at 1 h – and also delayed 24 h after sample taking, indicating that this topical steroid acts more profoundly on intestinal eosinophil function than on that of mucosal mast cells of the gut.

Ulcerative colitis

Release of mast cell tryptase as parameter of mast cell function

The rates of spontaneous and anti-IgE-induced T release in UC are given in Table 2. Overall, T secretion in UC was found to be slightly increased compared to GMA; however, in contrast to GMA, only spontaneous T secretion was slightly inhibited by budesonide, while the anti-IgE-induced T secretion appeared not to respond to budesonide. However, in UC, anti-IgE used in a concentration of 1/40 dilution (Sigma, Munich, Germany) appeared not to be a similarly effective functional trigger for mast cells as observed for eosinophils. This may indicate that mast cells in UC have already been degranulated *in vivo* by other stimuli[1,2,6], that other optimal anti-IgE concentrations may be needed or, at least, that the immunological activation process of the crosslinking anti-IgE antibody is not budesonide-sensitive in mast cells of UC, perhaps due to another or more severe immune up-regulation of mast cells function by the cytokine network.

Release of ECP as parameter of eosinophil function

The rates of spontaneous and anti-IgE-induced ECP release in UC are given in Table 3. As observed for the secretion of mast cell T, UC showed a substantially higher rate of ECP secretion than GMA. Spontaneous ECP secretion was therefore inhibited to a greater extent than T secretion in GMA by budesonide. In addition, anti-IgE stimulation in UC was found to be ineffective compared to ECP secretion in GMA in the presence of anti-IgE, again favouring the hypothesis that intestinal effector cells in UC may be regulated in another way than in GMA, may have required other optimal anti-IgE concentrations, or may have stimuli other than IgE-directed antibodies, or that they have already been degranulated *in vivo*[1,2,6].

DISCUSSION

When comparing the effect of budesonide on the secretory activity of human intestinal mast cells and eosinophils of living human tissue samples, the inhibitory effect of budesonide is more pronounced on eosinophil function than on mast cells. Although mucosa oxygenation was performed at two different time points with an immediate and delayed culture at day 1 and 2, the cultivation process was only 24 h and mast cell function should also be studied after longer incubation intervals in future, as steroids may exhibit their intracellular messages even after a longer incubation period.

Despite these restrictions the rapid inhibitory effect of budesonide on intestinal eosinophils is striking. Similar pathophysiological observations have been made in asthma bronchiale, a disease condition which is very similar to food allergy, as mast cells and eosinophils have been found to be predominant pathophysiological players in both these disease states which became activated by T-helper-2 cells. Thus GMA resembles asthma bronchiale more immunologically than UC. In so far as the pronounced inhibitory effect of budesonide on intestinal eosinophils in

GMA may be explained by a similar immunopathogenesis. In GMA, budesonide was found to inhibit both spontaneous and anti-IgE-induced ECP secretion with an impressive immediate and delayed effect, while in UC only spontaneous ECP secretion was influenced.

Thus the use of budesonide in UC may have an impact on spontaneous eosinophil activity, while in GMA therapeutic studies with budesonide may be warranted to down-regulate eosinophil function basically, but also to reduce effector cell degranulation after an inadvertent food antigen ingestion. The beneficial effect of budesonide on intestinal eosinophils in GMA may thus favour the use of this topically active steroid in patients with chronic relapsing severe GMA in whom polyvalent antigen sensitizations are present and/or allergen avoidance as primary treatment choice does not work, with predominant eosinophil activation in serum or mucosa and perhaps in patients with eosinophil gastroenteritis.

Although, in food allergy no systematic studies with budesonide have been performed until now, a first beneficial report was published in a patient with eosinophilic gastroenteritis[12]. The effect of budesonide in this steroid-dependent patient may be explained, at least in part, with these observed striking experimental findings of budesonide on intestinal eosinophil function, as eosinophilic gastroenteritis is a well-known condition in which activity is strongly correlated with eosinophil number, degranulation rate and function. Thus, budesonide appears to have the potential to exert beneficial effects in several intestinal disorders which are characterized by an up-regulation of eosinophil granulocytes, e.g. food hypersensitivity, eosinophilic gastroenteritis or microscopic, colitis etc.

References

1. Balazs M, Illyes G, Vadasz G. Mast cells in ulcerative colitis. Quantitative and ultrastructural studies. Virchows Arch B Cell Pathol. 1989;57:353–60.
2. Rampton DS, Murdoch RD, Sladen GE. Rectal mucosal histamine release in ulcerative colitis. Clin Sci. 1980;59:389–91.
3. Knutson L, Ahrenstedt O, Odlind B, Hallgren R. The jejunal secretion of histamine is increased in active Crohn's disease. Gastroenterology. 1990;98:849–54.
4. Raithel M, Hochberger J, Hahn EG. Effect of colonoscopy-premedication containing diazepam and pethidine on the release of mast cell mediators from gut mucosal samples. Endoscopy. 1995;27:415–23.
5. Raithel M, Ulrich P, Pacurara A, Winterkamp S, Hochberger J, Hahn EG. Release of mast cell tryptase from human colorectal mucosa in inflammatory bowel disease. Scand J Gastroenterol. 2001;36:174–9.
6. Stenton GR, Vliagoftis H, Befus D. Role of intestinal mast cells in modulating gastrointestinal pathopyhsiology. Ann Allergy Asthma Immunol. 1998;81:1–11.
7. Enander I, Matsson P, Nystrand J et al. A new radioimmunoassay for human mast cell tryptase using monoclonal antibodies. J Immunol Methods. 1991;138:39–46.
8. Alter CS, Schwartz LB. Tryptase: an indicator of mast cell mediated allergic reactions. In: Spector L, editor. Provocative Challenge Procedures: Background and Methodology. Mount Kisco NY: Futura, 1989:167–83.
9. Schwab D, Raithel M, Klein P et al. Immunoglobulin E and eosinophilic cationic protein in segmental lavage fluid of the small and large bowel identifies patients with food allergy. Am J Gastroenterol. 2001;96:508–14.
10. Raithel M, Weidenhiller M, Schwab D, Winterkamp S, Hahn EG. Pancreatic enzymes: a new group of antiallergic drugs? Inflamm Res. 2002;51(Suppl. 1): S13–14.

11. Weidenhiller M, Traenkner A, Schwab D, Hahn EG, Raithel M. Different kinetics of mediator release can be detected during allergic reactions after oral provocation (double blind placebo-controlled food challenge). Inflamm Res. 2002;51(Suppl. 1): 29–30.
12. Tan ACITL, Kruimel JW, Naber THJ. Eosinophilic gastroenteritis treated with non-enteric-coated budesonide tablets. Eur J Gastroenterol Hepatol. 2001;13:425–7.

9
Use of oral budesonide in paediatric inflammatory bowel disease

A. LEVINE

Successful treatment of Crohn's disease (CD) requires therapeutic options that will achieve and maintain remission of the disease. These are achieved medically initially with medications and nutritional therapy. Medications that are useful for achieving remission may not be as useful for maintaining remission and vice-versa. A drawback associated with medical therapy for active CD to date is the observation that medications with the greatest potential to achieve remission also carry the highest risks for side-effects. Therapy of active disease in both paediatric and adult patients has traditionally utilized a stepwise approach. Patients with milder disease are often treated initially with the medications that are less efficient, but have fewer side-effects, while patients with more severe disease are treated with medications that induce higher remission rates, but have more severe side-effects.

Treatment strategies in paediatric patients are not much different from the strategies used in adults, though two issues may be different and affect these strategies[1]. The first issue is the effect of disease activity and medications on growth. Active disease and conventional corticosteroids can inhibit growth and bone mineral density, during a critical period when maximal height velocity and bone mineral accretion are at their maximum. Inhibition of either process during this period may expose children to irreversible loss of final height or of peak bone mineral density[2,3]. The second important issue is side-effects. Both psychological and pathophysiological side-effects related to medications, and especially to corticosteroids, may cause severe problems related to distorted body image, non-compliance or failure to report disease activity. Use of systemic corticosteroids in children is a source of contention[1].

Oral budesonide is a potent steroid that undergoes extensive first-pass metabolism to nearly inactive metabolites 6-hydroxybudesonide and 16-hydroxy-prednisolone. It has a systemic bioavailability of about 10%, and has a significantly higher affinity for the glucocorticoid receptor[4]. Many studies have shown that remission rates of about 50% can be expected in adults with appropriately located active CD[5–9]. Remission rates have been shown to be superior to those achieved by mesalamine, but with fewer side-effects and a superior quality of life[10]. Remission rates are equal to, or inferior to, conventional oral corticosteroids, again with fewer side-effects[9]. Subgroup analysis has shown that, for patients with mild disease activity, budesonide might have remission rates equivalent to those of prednisone therapy[11].

Three studies to date have addressed the issue of oral budesonide in paediatric CD. Levine et al.[12] evaluated 120 paediatric patients with active disease treated with either prednisone 40 mg/day or budesonide 9 mg/day. Inclusion criteria included a paediatric Crohn's disease activity index of 12.5–40. Patients were matched for age, gender and site of disease. They were evaluated for remission rate, remission after failing previous first-line therapy, and parameters associated with increased likelihood of remission. Four findings from this study were of significance. The first was that oral prednisone caused a higher remission rate than oral budesonide. Among children treated with budesonide, 48% achieved remission, in comparison to 77% of the children treated with prednisone ($p = 0.001$). Remission with prednisone occurred in 73% of children who failed to achieve remission with budesonide. In addition, patients responding to budesonide had significantly milder disease in comparison to non-responders who remitted with prednisone. The second conclusion was that budesonide appeared to be superior to mesalamine. Among patients who had failed previous medical therapy with mesalamine, 59% achieved remission with budesonide 9 mg/day. The third conclusion was that step-up therapy with budesonide, followed by prednisone if budesonide failed, led to a similar remission rate to those patients treated with prednisone alone. This supports the notion that step-up therapy can lead to avoidance of prednisone in approximately 50% of patients with mild to moderate active disease, without compromising likelihood of remission. The fourth conclusion was that failure to respond to budesonide was statistically correlated with measures of severity or activity, but not distal colonic involvement.

The second study was a prospective randomized controlled study comparing oral budesonide to oral prednisone for mild to moderate active disease, defined as before[13]. This study was underpowered to evaluate remission rates due to under-enrollment in the prednisone arm. The endpoints were remission rates (at 12 weeks), and side-effects. Data from this study are portrayed in Tables 1 and 2. The remission rate for budesonide in this study was 47%, not significantly different from prednisone. Side-effects occurred in 32% and 71% of patients treated with budesonide and prednisone, respectively ($p < 0.05$). Severity of cosmetic side-effects was significantly lower in patients treated with budesonide ($p < 0.01$).

These studies have shown that similar remission rates can be achieved in children and adolescents, with fewer and less significant side-effects than conventional steroids. These data suggest that in children and adolescents with

Table 1 Response to budesonide and prednisone at week 12, compared to baseline

	Budesonide *Group 1*	*Prednisone* *Group 2*
Remission rate	9/19 (47%)	7/14 (50%)
Drop in PCDAI (points)	9.3 ± 14.8	13.4 ± 10.6
Weight gain (kg)	1.6 ± 2.5	3.7 ± 3.0*

*$p < 0.05$

Table 2 Comparison of side-effects between oral budesonide and prednisone

Parameter	Budesonide Group 1	Prednisone Group 2
Total side-effects (%)	6/19 (31.6)	10.14 (71.4)*
Significant effects (%)	1/19 (7.7)	3/13 (21)
Cosmetic severity score (mean $\pm$ SD)	0.5 ± 0.8	1.68 ± 1.6**

*$p < 0.05$; **$p < 0.01$

appropriately located mild to moderate disease, budesonide should be considered before conventional steroids, and may replace mesalamine in the future as a first-line drug. Issues that have not been resolved include the optimal dose in paediatrics, and the use of budesonide in patients with colonic involvement. These issues are currently being addressed in a prospective double-blind trial that is already under way.

Acknowledgements

We thank Mona Boaz PhD for her help with the statistical analysis.

References

1. Levine A, Milo T, Buller H, Markowitz J. Consensus and controversy in the management of pediatric Crohn's disease: an international survey. J Pediatr Gastroenterol Nutr. 2003;36:464–9.
2. Semeao EJ, Jawad AF, Stouffer NO, Zemel BS, Picolli DA, Stallings VA. Risk factors for low bone mineral density in children and young adults with Crohn's disease. J Pediatr. 1999;135:593–600.
3. Gokhale R, Favus M, Karrison T, Sutton M, Rich B, Kirschner B. Bone mineral density assessment in children with inflammatory bowel disease. Gastroenterology. 1998;114:902–11.
4. Spencer CM, McTavish D. Budesonide: a review of its pharmacological properties and therapeutic efficacy in inflammatory bowel disease. Drugs. 1995;50:854–72.
5. Thomsen OO, Cortot A, Jewell D et al. A comparison of budesonide and mesalamine for active Crohn's disease. International budesonide–mesalamine study group. N Engl J Med. 1998;339:370–4.
6. Bar-Meir S, Chowers Y, Lavy A et al. Budesonide versus prednisone in the treatment of active Crohn's disease. Gastroenterology. 1998;115:835–40.
7. Campieri M, Ferguson A, Doe W et al. Oral budesonide is as effective as oral prednisolone in active Crohn's disease. Gut. 1997;41:209–14.
8. Rutgeerts P, Lofberg R, Malchow H et al. A comparison of budesonide with prednisolone for active Crohn's disease. N Engl J Med. 1994;331:842–5.
9. Papi C, Luchetti R, Gili L et al. Budesonide in the treatment of Crohn's disease: a meta-analysis. Aliment Pharmacol Ther. 2000;14:1419–28.
10. Thomsen OO, Cortot A, Jewel D et al. Budesonide and mesalazine in active Crohn's disease: a comparison of the effects on quality of life. Am J Gastroenterol. 2002;97:649–53.
11. Kane Schoenfeld P, Sandborn WJ, Tremaine W, Hofer T, Feagan BG. The effectiveness of budesonide therapy for Crohn's disease. Aliment Pharmacol Ther. 2002;16:1509–17.
12. Levine A, Broide E, Stein M et al. Evaluation of oral budesonide for treatment of mild and moderate exacerbations of Crohn's disease in children. J Pediatr. 2002;140:75–80.13.
13 Levine A, Weizman Z, Shamir R et al. A comparison of budesonide and prednisone for the treatment of active pediatric Crohn's disease. J Pediatr Gastroenterol Nutr. 2003;36:248–52.

10
The therapeutic potential of budesonide for oral mucosal diseases

S. ELAD, R. OR, A. HAVIV and M. Y. SHAPIRA

BACKGROUND

Oral mucosal diseases consist of a wide range of pathologies[1]. They can be grouped into two main classes. The first class is composed of systemic diseases with oral manifestations, the second group consists of isolated oral mucosal lesions. This classification is fundamental to understanding of principles of topical oral budesonide treatment.

The broad spectrum of diagnoses in the group of systemic diseases with oral manifestations includes vesiculobullous diseases and ulcerative conditions. The short list that follows emphasizes the scope of the clinical challenge: Behçet's syndrome, Crohn's disease, erythema multiforme, Stevens Johnson syndrome, drug reactions, lupus erythematosus, graft-versus-host disease (GvHD), pemphigus vulgaris, paraneoplastic pemphigus, cicatrical pemphigoid, bullous pemphigoid, dermatitis herpetiformis and epidermolysis bullosa. Two isolated oral mucosal ulcerative diseases are dominant in the second group: aphthous ulcers/recurrent aphthous ulcers (RAU) and lichen planus. These diagnoses are fairly common. RAU is reported to have a prevalence of up to 66 000 out of 100 000 people[2]. Lichen planus affects 200–2200 out of 100 000 people[3].

Any of the above-mentioned diagnoses may cause dramatic lesions in the oral cavity, affecting oral function and quality of life.

These pathologies have immunological and inflammatory components; therefore the overall treatment approach for these lesions includes anti-inflammatory agents as well as immunomodulators. Due to the many similarities and differences in the above-mentioned pathologies a generalized description of treatment options will be presented here.

Current first-line treatment is based on steroidal preparations. Among the well-known steroidal preparations are triamcinolone acetonide, flucinonide and dexamethasone[2]. Second-line treatments include immunomodulators such as levamisole, colchicine, azathioprine, dapsone, thalidomide, azelastine, cyclosporin, amlexanax and 5-aminosalicyclic acid[2].

Despite the systemic nature of some of these conditions oral topical treatment is needed in most patients. There are two main reasons for oral topical treatment:

first, oral lesions are often refractory to systemic treatment; secondly, when the oral mucosa is the only site involved, topical treatment may prevent the severe side-effects associated with systemic treatments.

As mentioned above, topical steroidal preparations are among the first-line treatments for these diseases. Unfortunately there is no commercially available preparation of the most potent topical steroidal preparation, dexamethasone.

The topical use of immunomodulators such as azathioprine, cyclosporin and FK506 has not been officially approved. Accordingly, evidence of the beneficial effects of these drugs can be gleaned only from clinical trials at universities and hospitals.

THE SELECTION OF BUDESONIDE

Budesonide has several characteristics that make topical mucosal use appropriate. It possesses a high ratio of topical to systemic activity compared with other corticosteroids such as beclomethasone dipropionate and prednisolone[4]. Budesonide undergoes rapid inactivation by biotransformation in the liver[4,5] producing low-potency metabolites[6]. A very low risk of systemic side-effects exists with the recommended dosage for treatment of mucous membranes[5,7,8].

Budesonide is well tolerated during long-term treatments[9]. Although a dose–response relationship with plasma cortisol concentration has been documented, little or no suppression of adrenal function occurs during treatment at recommended dosages. Furthermore its high anti-inflammatory effect and strong affinity for corticosteroid receptors, relative to other steroids, accentuate its potency for treatment of oral GvHD[6,10].

Budesonide is used safely and successfully in bronchial asthma, allergic rhinitis[11] and chronic inflammatory bowel disease[12,13]. Recently budesonide was assessed for use as a topical treatment for acute intestinal GvHD[14]. Bertz et al. concluded that budesonide may be effective for this condition[14]. Based on these results we carried out a preliminary study to evaluate the efficacy of budesonide for oral mucosal GvHD.

CLINICAL EXPERIENCE

The study population consisted of 12 patients post-bone marrow transplantation (BMT) with either severe oral steroid-resistant chronic GvHD or contraindications to systemic steroids. Patients were instructed to rinse their mouths with budesonide mouthwash for 15 min, three times a day, for 2 weeks. They were examined 2 weeks later, and mucosal response was evaluated. During this time systemic immunosuppressant doses were not changed.

Table 1 summarizes the data of the first group of patients treated with topical oral budesonide[15]. Among the 12 patients treated, five were classified as extensive GvHD, and seven as limited GvHD. On average they were 1 year post-BMT. All were treated with systemic prednisone and other immunomodulators. Some patients used topical treatments such as dexamethasone mouthwash; however, additional treatment was still required.

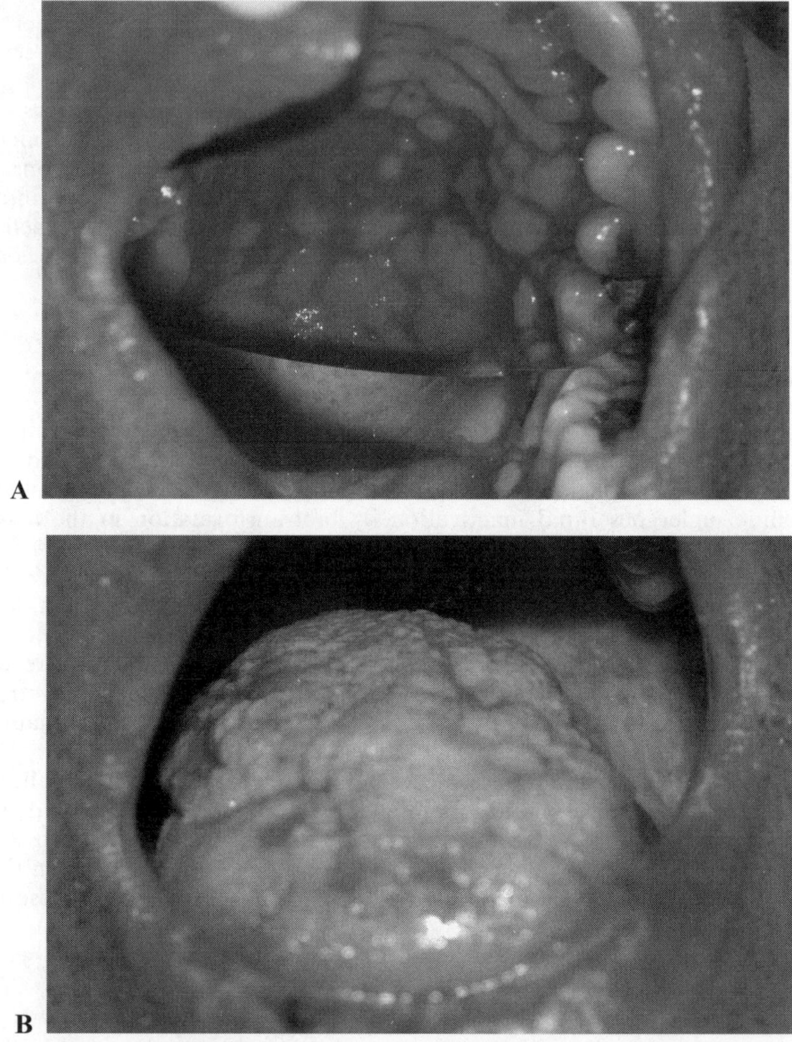

Figure 1 A 39-year-old patient diagnosed with acute myelogenous leukaemia, status post bone marrow transplantation in 1999. He suffers from severe chronic oral GvHD and was treated with 1 mg/kg prednisone, cyclosporin and azathioprine, with no improvement. Intra-oral examination revealed extensive erythematous and ulcerative lesions. (**A**) palatal view; (**B**) dorsum of the tongue

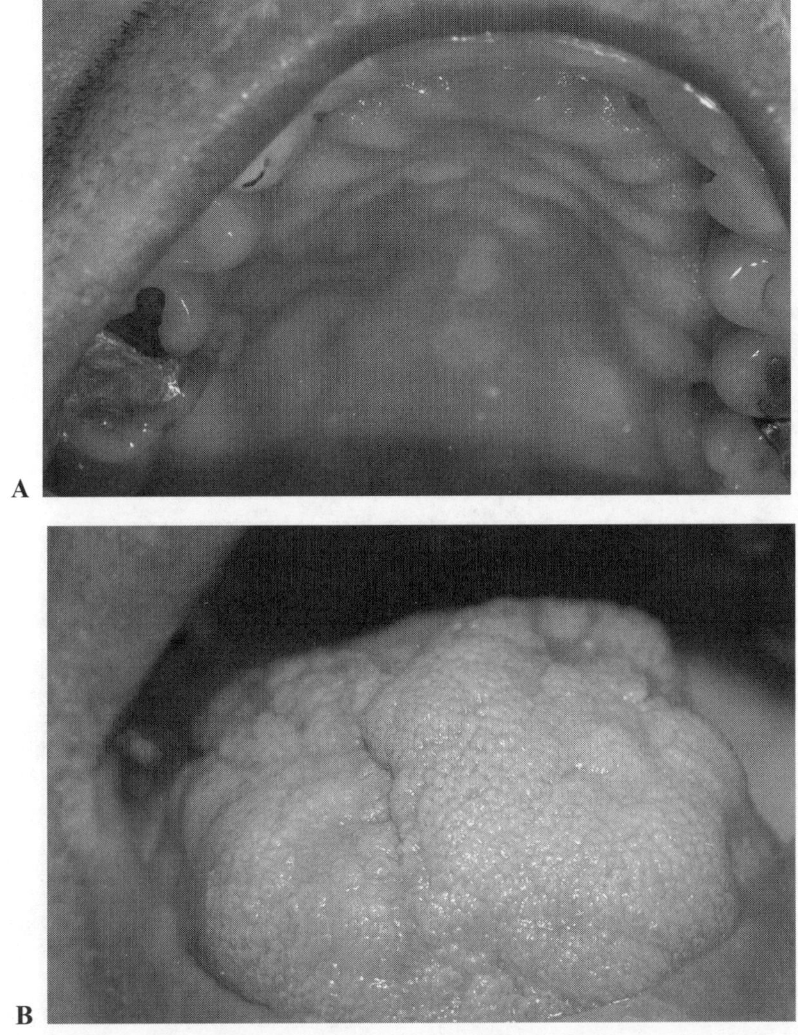

Figure 2 Two weeks after initiation of budesonide oral mouthwashes, marked reduction in erythematous and ulcerative lesions. (**A**) palatal view; (**B**) dorsum of the tongue

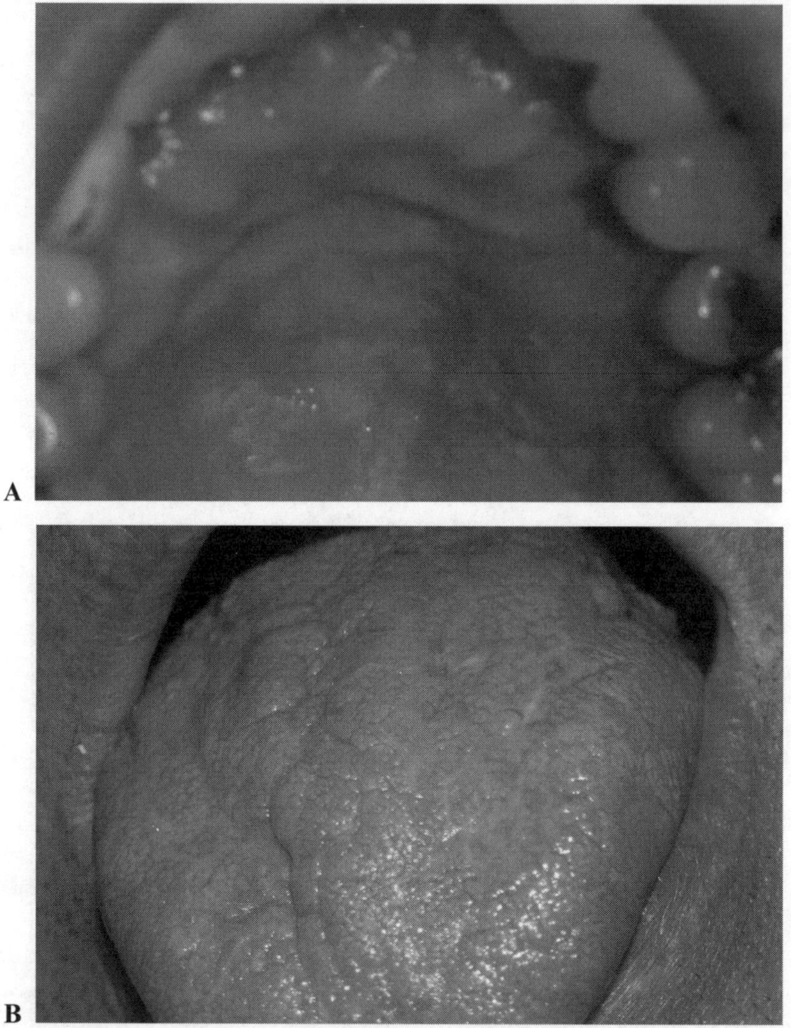

Figure 3 After 3 months, further improvement was noted. No ulcerations were seen. (**A**) palatal view: a superficial erosion at site of the most severe ulceration was noted; (**B**) dorsum of the tongue

Table 1 Summary of patient characteristics and previous treatments

Patient no.	Age (years)	Indication for HSCT	GvHD type	GvHD onset	GvHD severity	Systemic		Oral topical	
						Prednisone (mg/kg per day)	Other	Dexa	Other
1	48	CML	Chronic	Progressive	Extensive	2	CsP, T, A	+	–
2	54	NHL	Chronic	De novo	Limited	0.5	CsP	+	Ret., UVB
3	40	APL	Chronic	Progressive	Extensive	0.75	CsP	+	UVB
4	54	NHL	Chronic	De novo	Extensive	–	CsP, A	+	–
5	46	CML	Chronic	Progressive	Limited	–	T, A	–	–
6	34	AML	Chronic	Progressive	Limited	0.75	CsP	+	–
7	23	AML	Chronic	Progressive	Extensive	0.75	MTX, T, A	+	UVB
8	26	ALL	Chronic	De novo	Extensive	0.2	CsP	+	–
9	38	AML	Chronic	Progressive	Limited	1	CsP, A	–	–
10	48	CML	Chronic	De novo	Limited	0.4	CsP, A	–	–
11	48	NHL	Chronic	De novo	Limited	–	CsP	–	–
12	21	MDS	Chronic	De novo	Limited	–	CsP	–	–

CML, chronic myelogenous leukaemia; NHL, non-Hodgkin's lymphoma; APL, acute promyelocytic leukaemia; AML, acute myelogenous leukaemia; CsP, cyclosporin A; Dexa, dexamethasone mouthwash; T, thalidomide; A, azathioprine; MTX, methotrexate; Ret, Retinoids; UVB, ultraviolet B; MDS, myelodysplastic syndrome; HSCT, haematopoietic stem cell transplantation; GvHD, graft-versus-host disease

In order to evaluate the response to budesonide treatment we defined a five-level scale, where 'no response' is 'no change in the oral GvHD signs'; 'mild response' is 'a limited reduction of the involved mucosal surface area, or early healing of ulcerated lesions'; 'moderate response' is 'a reduction of the involved mucosal surface area, or incomplete healing of ulcerated lesions, or a reduction of the severity of the erythema'; 'good response' is 'a marked reduction of the involved mucosal surface area, healing of ulcerated lesions, and a reduction of the severity of the erythema'; and 'complete response' is 'a complete resolution of the oral GvHD'.

Budesonide topical treatment did not cause any major systemic side-effects. A local burning sensation was reported in one case. All patients reported subjective improvements. The examiner recorded objective responses and seven of the 12 patients were scored as having a good to complete response[16]. The mean lag time to initial response was 14 days. Gradual reduction of prednisone and cyclosporin doses commenced as early as 2 weeks following the initiation of budesonide mouthwashes.

At long-term follow-up we noted high patient compliance. Doses were adjusted from once to three times daily during the follow-up period according to fluctuations in oral manifestations.

Oral candidiasis was observed in two patients after 6 months of daily budesonide mouthwashes; this was not surprising as oral candidiasis is a well-known complication of topical steroid treatment. In both patients the candidiasis responded well to topical antifungal agents.

In contrast to GvHD, which is a systemic disease, occurring in post-BMT patients, RAU is an inflammatory condition limited to the oral mucosa.

Treating a patient suffering from RAU enabled us to follow the response of RAU to budesonide topical treatment over time, and to compare it to an untreated lesion in the same patient. We tried two modes of application: spraying directly on the lesion and applying gauze soaked with budesonide on the localized lesion. The preliminary findings suggest the aphthae healed faster with budesonide treatment. In addition, the earlier the patient begins treatment the greater the effect of budesonide on healing.

With daily budesonide application the patient reported relief of pain prior to complete healing.

In summary, budesonide may be suitable for topical use. Budesonide was suggested to be beneficial in the management of localized disease (RAU) and oral manifestations of a systemic disease (GvHD). The treatment is simple, although an improved mode of application is required for topical use. Additionally, side-effects were uncommon, with oral candidiasis seen in only two patients after long-term use, and easily controlled with topical antifungals.

It is clear from these preliminary studies that budesonide has great potential, and that large-scale studies comparing budesonide to other steroids are warranted. We have demonstrated two potential patient groups that would benefit from topical treatment, and believe that the number of oral mucosal lesions managed with topical budesonide will increase as more research is undertaken.

References

1. Regezi JA, Sciubba JJ, editors. Oral Pathology. Clinical–Pathologic Correlations, 3rd edn. Philadelphia, PA: Saunders, 2000.
2. Porter SR, Scully C, Pederson A. Recurrent aphthous stomatitis. Crit Rev Oral Biol Med. 1998;9:306–21.
3. Neville BW, Damm DD, Allen CM, Bouquot JE, editors. Oral and Maxillofacial Pathology. Philadelphia, PA: Saunders, 1995.
4. Rutgeerts P, Lofberg R, Malchow H et al. A comparison of budesonide with prednisolone for active Crohn's disease. N Engl J Med. 1994;331:842–5.
5. Spencer CM, McTravish D. Budesonide. A review of its pharmacological properties and therapeutic efficacy in inflammatory bowel disease. Drugs. 1991;50:854–72.
6. Thalen A, Brattsand R, Andersson PH. Development of glucocorticosteroids with enhanced ratio between topical and systemic effects. Acta Derm Venereol. 1989;69(Suppl.):11–19.
7. Hellers G, Cortot A, Jewell D et al. Oral budesonide for prevention of postsurgical recurrence in Crohn's disease. IOIBD Budesonide Study Group. Gastroenterology. 1999;116:294–300.
8. Lofberg R, Danielsson A, Suhr O et al. Oral budesonide versus prednisolone in patients with active extensive and left sided ulcerative colitis. Gastroenterology. 1996;110:1713–18.
9. Johasson G, Carlsen KH, Jonasson C, Mowinckel P. Low-dose inhaled budesonide once or twice daily for 27 months in children with mild asthma. Allergy. 2000;55:740–8.
10. Dahlberg E, Thalen A, Brattsand R et al. Correlation between chemical structure, receptor binding, and biological activity in some novel, highly active, 16α,17α-acetal-substituted glucocorticoids. Mol Pharmacol. 1984;25:70–8.
11. Brogdan RN, McTravish D. Budesonide. An updated review of its pharmacological properties and therapeutic effects in asthma and rhinitis. Drugs. 1992;44:375–407.
12. Thomson ABR, Sadowski D, Jenkins R, Wild G. Budesonide in the management of patients with Crohn's disease. Can J Gasteroenterol. 1997;11:255–60.
13. Danielson A. Treatment of distal ulcerative colitis with non-systemic corticosteroid enemas. Scand J Gastroenterol. 1996;31:945–53.
14. Bertz H, Afting M, Kreisel W, Duffner U, Greinwald R, Finke J. Feasibility and response to budesoinde as topical corticosteroid therapy for acute intestinal GVHD. Bone Marrow Transplant. 1999;24:1185–9.
15. Elad S, Or R, Garfunkel AA, Shapira MY. Budesonide: a novel treatment for oral chronic graft versus host disease. Oral Surg Oral Med Oral Pathol Oral Radiol Endod. 2003;95:308–11.

Section III
Potential use of budesonide after surgical interventions and in patients with oncological complications

11
Potential use of budesonide after surgical interventions and in patients with oncological complications – functional improvement in patients with ileostomy

K.-W. ECKER

INTRODUCTION

Under normal conditions the intestinal mucosa absorbs about 8–9 L of water over 24 h; only 100 ml are excreted with the faeces. After proctocolectomy and ileostomy the intestinal output can be estimated according to the basic disease with about 300–500 ml in familial adenomatous polyposis (FAP), 400–800 ml in ulcerative colitis (UC) and 600–1200 ml in Crohn's disease (CD). Especially after ileal resection because of CD, a so-called high intestinal output syndrome with an ileal output of more than 1000 ml can often be observed. While an ileostoma output of 300–700 ml per day may be tolerated by patients[1], higher outputs result in chronic dehydration, electrolyte disturbances, neurological and psychiatric symptoms, severely reducing the patient's quality of life.

In some patients the high intestinal output syndrome may be due to a co-resection of the ileum; in others the function of the remaining intestinal mucosa may be impaired. In most cases both factors seem to be causative. In inflammatory bowel disease (IBD) an impairment of intestinal adaptation occurs more often in patients with CD than in those with UC. The therapeutic efficacy of approaches aimed at reducing ileostomy output by motility-influencing agents such as loperamide, or inhibition of secretion by growth hormones (somatostatin), is limited[2–5]. Therefore data from experimental studies showing positive effects of corticoids on epithelial transport function[6,7] and findings in patients with IBD[8] may open a new therapy option. The effects of glucocorticoids on intestinal output appear quickly and are separate from the anti-inflammatory effects of these agents. Two studies were performed to evaluate the beneficial effect of topical budesonide.

METHODS

In study 1[9] the influence on ileostoma output was quantified at short-term treatment in CD patients with high ileostomal output syndrome after ileostomy[1]. In the second study the stability of the effect and the reproducibility was analysed under long-term treatment. Methods and patients of the two studies are summarized in Table 1. Both studies complied with the principles of the Helsinki Declaration and were approved by the ethics committee of the medical association of the Saarland, Germany.

STUDY 1

In study 1[9] the effect of oral budesonide (3×3 mg daily for 8 days) on the intestinal output of ileostomy patients with CD in remission after exclusion of any inflammatory activity was analysed. The ileostomy output at baseline was measured by self-report under normal dietary conditions and no fluid intake restrictions, and exceeded 1000 ml per day. Treatment with corticosteroids was prohibited during the 4 weeks preceding entry to the study. Exclusion criteria included use of substances affecting absorption, intestinal motility or the measurement methods used in this investigation; other severe diseases decreasing life expectancy; pregnancy, lactation or unreliable contraception; and contra-indications for corticoid treatment. For evaluation, two groups were formed: group A (ileal resection length 0–20 cm) and group B (ileal resection length >20 cm).

Study performance

The performance schedule of the study is summarized in Figure 1. The standard diet prior to beginning treatment and on the last day of medication was defined as a 2000 kcal ($\approx 8\,000\,000$ J) diet (breakfast, 500 kcal $\approx 2\,000\,000$ J; lunch, 1000 kcal $\approx 4\,000\,000$ J; dinner, 500 kcal $\approx 2\,000\,000$ J) and 2000 ml of tea. Patients were instructed to drink 200 ml at each meal, with 1100 ml to be consumed in 100-ml portions during the day at hourly intervals. The remaining 300 ml were to be consumed during the night according to demand. Emptying of ileostomy bags was counted at 12-h intervals, and stool volume was determined by a graduated measure as well as by taking stool weights.

The following laboratory data were determined on day $-1/0$ prior to beginning treatment and on day $8/9$ after termination of treatment: complete blood count (days -1, 8 and 9), erythrocyte sedimentation rate (1 h/2 h), serum protein (total serum protein, protein electrophoresis, C-reactive protein, serum immunoglobulin A, immunoglobulin G, immunoglobulin M), electrolytes (sodium, potassium, chloride, phosphate), renal parameters (creatinine, urea) and liver enzymes (glutamate oxalo-acetate transaminase, glutamate pyruvate transaminase, gamma glutamyl transferase, alkaline phosphatase).

At endoscopy the mucosa was assessed macroscopically and scored at 10 cm intervals to the following stages: 0 = mucosa normal; 1 = mucosa blushed, inflamed without lesions; 2 = aphthae, fissures, small ulcers; 3 = deep ulcers,

Table 1 Methods and patients of two studies on the effect of topical budesonide on high intestinal output syndrome in patients with ileostomy for Crohn's disease

	Study 1	Study 2
Design	Prospective, monocentric, placebo controlled, double-blind, matched-pair randomization	Open, monocentric, intra-individual comparison after withdrawal and re-exposure
Inclusion criteria	Intestinal output > 1000 ml/24 h, no acute inflammation, informed consent	Intestinal output > 1000 ml/24 h no active inflammation, treatment of at least 4 weeks before start of study
Population		
No.	2×20 patients	22 patients
Age	18–60 years	40.6 ± 6.1 years (18–70 years)
Gender	Male (15), female (25)	Male (7), female (16)
Time at start of treatment	Time since ileostoma construction 17–154 months	Pre-treatment 36.7 months
Ileal resection lengths	0–10 cm: $n = 2 \times 5$ 11–20 cm: $n = 2 \times 4$ 21–30 cm: $n = 2 \times 2$ > 30 cm: $n = 2 \times 9$	36.3 ± 30.2 cm

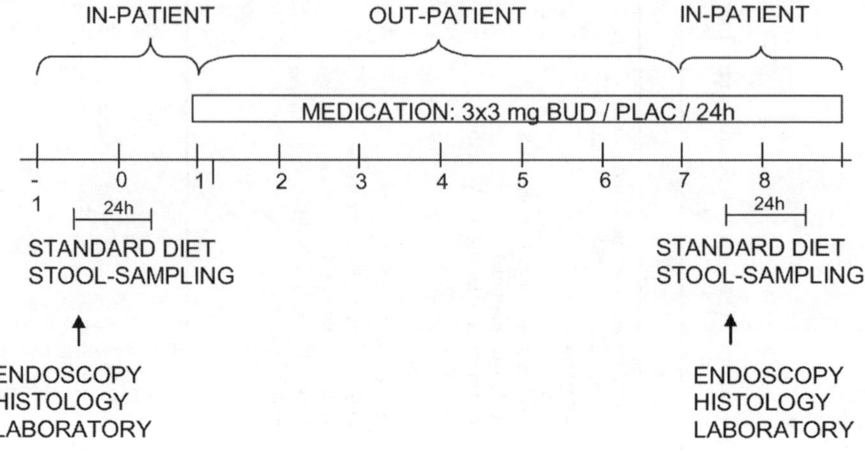

Figure 1 Performance schedule of study 1 (in weeks). BUD = budesonide, PLAC = placebo

extended ulcers, stenoses, fistular openings. Biopsies taken during ileoscopy were analysed histologically at light microscopy. Histological results were assigned to stages 0 = normal, no inflammatory changes; 1 = small inflammatory changes without mucosa defects; 2 = inflammatory changes with granular infiltration and mucosa defects; 3 = dense inflammatory infiltrates in all biopsies as well as mucosal erosions and ulcerations.

Statistics

Response to treatment was determined by an intra-individual comparison of intestinal output before and after 8 days of treatment. A >25% reduction in intestinal output during treatment was defined as response. The response rate was evaluated on the base of the per-protocol analysis ($n = 2 \times 20$).

A difference in response rates between budesonide and placebo of at least 50% was assumed to be of clinical relevance. According to this assumption a sample size of 13–16 patients per group was calculated using the 'N' program (IDV – Institut für Datenanalyse und Versuchsplanung, Gauting).

The response rate was confirmed by the one-sided Fisher exact test (α-level, 5%). Subgroups were analysed by the two-sided Fisher exact test and by interpretation of the two-fold one-sided p-value. Differences in volume and weight of ileostomy output between the treatment groups were analysed by the Wilcoxon–Mann–Whitney U-test.

Results

Both patient groups were comparable in terms of demographic, surgical history, general health, prior medication and other relevant parameters. Under conditions of normal nutrition all patients reported ileostomy output exceeding 1000 ml/day (self-report). All patients were included in the statistical evaluation.

Response rates

In the budesonide group 60% (12/20) of patients showed a response, defined as reduction of intestinal output by $>25\%$. No patient of the placebo group responded to the treatment based on this criterion. The difference was statistically significant ($p<0.0001$) with calculated 95% confidence intervals for the probability to show a response of 36.1–80.9% for budesonide and 0–16.8% for placebo. This confirmed the main aim of the study with a significance level of $<1\%$ and a power of $>80\%$ (99.8%).

In the subgroups the response rates to budesonide treatment in patients with ileal resection lengths of $\leqslant 20$ cm and >20 cm were 88.9% (8/9 patients, subgroup A) and 36.4% (4/11 patients, subgroup B). The difference was significant at the 5% level ($p = 0.0498$). Corresponding 95% confidence intervals were 51.8–99.7% ($\leqslant 20$ cm) and 10.9–69.2% (>20 cm), respectively.

Ileostomal output

The median absolute daily intestinal output in the budesonide group decreased from 1240 ml at baseline to 865 ml at final examination (30.2%), compared to a negligible decrease from 950 ml to 947.5 ml (0.3%) in the placebo group (Figure 2). In the budesonide group the median ileostomy output at baseline (1240 ml) was about one-third higher than in the placebo group (950 ml). This difference was not statistically significant in the Wilcoxon–Mann–Whitney U-test (exact two-sided p-value = 0.0751). This was mainly due to three patients in the budesonide group with extremely high output exceeding 2000 ml on day –1/0. Omitting these extreme values the median output was reduced to 1155 ml ($n =$ 17). The reduction of ileostomy output on day 8/9 was significantly higher in the budesonide group compared to placebo, irrespective of the higher or lower baseline value on day –1/0.

In the budesonide arm the subgroups of patients with resection lengths of $\leqslant 20$ cm or >20 cm showed a comparable absolute median reduction in ileostomy output of 400 ml and 405 ml, respectively. The baseline median ileostomy output of budesonide-treated patients with an ileal resection length $\leqslant 20$ cm (1020 ml) decreased by 39.2% to 620 ml. At an ileal resection length >20 cm the baseline output was higher (1645 ml) and decreased by 24.6% to 1240 ml (Figure 3). In the placebo group the median ileal output changed from 850 ml to 930 ml (increase by 9.4%) in patients with an ileal resection length of $\leqslant 20$ cm and remained nearly unchanged at an ileal resection length >20 cm (1115 ml vs. 1060 ml, –4.9%).

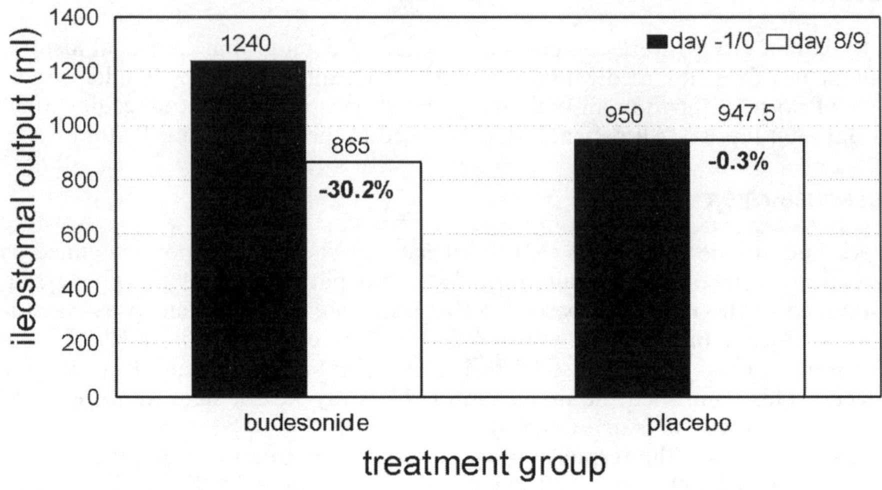

Figure 2   Median 24-h ileostomal output prior to beginning treatment (day –1/0) and at the end of treatment (day 8/9)

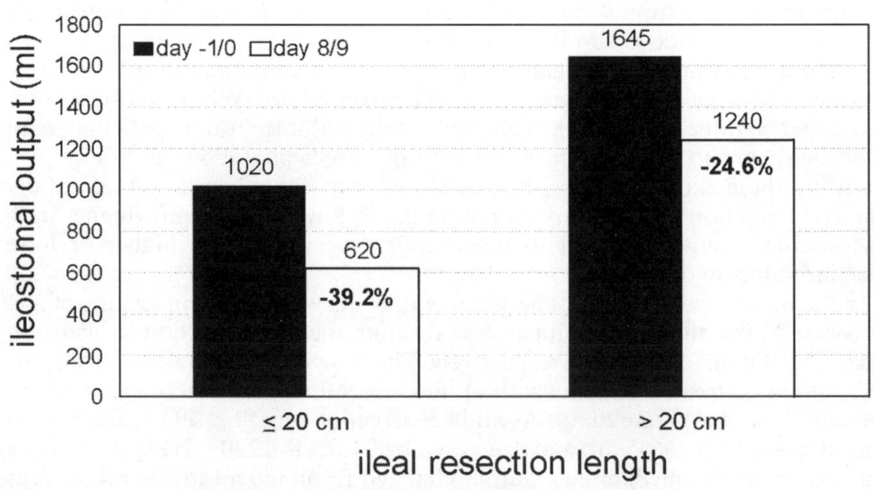

Figure 3   Median 24-h ileostomal output during budesonide treatment in subgroups with ileal resection length ⩽ 20 cm and ileal resection length > 20 cm

Inflammatory activity and other laboratory data

In most patients of both treatment groups neither macroscopic (endoscopy) nor microscopic (histopathology) examination revealed evidence of morphological changes consistent with inflammation. Haematological studies returned normal levels for both platelets and leucocytes before and after treatment in both the budesonide and the placebo groups. However, C-reactive protein was slightly increased before treatment in both groups, but showed normalization with both budesonide and placebo. In contrast the erythrocyte sedimentation rate showed a tendential increase during the treatment period both for the budesonide and the placebo groups. Serum protein, electrolytes and renal parameter were normal in both groups before and after treatment.

STUDY 2

In study 2 the long-term effect of budesonide was evaluated by rebound effects after withdrawal of budesonide and re-exposure. The basic data of the patients are listed in Table 1. All patients were under medication with 3×3 mg budesonide daily because of high intestinal output syndrome for at least 4 weeks: mean duration of pre-treatment was 36.7 ± 45.3 weeks, 12 patients had a history of budesonide treatment (3×3 mg daily) of at least 4 up to 10 weeks, 11 patients had been treated with budesonide at least 20 weeks before the study started (maximum 155 weeks). The weight of the patients measured remained stable during the trial.

Study performance

The performance schedule of the study is shown in Figure 4. The treatment was performed under outpatient conditions. In phase 1 (1 week, day $1-7 \pm 1$), the patients took 3×3 mg budesonide (morning, noon, evening) as they did previously. In phase 2 (4 weeks, day $8-35 \pm 1$), budesonide was omitted (withdrawal phase), and in phase 3 (1 week, day $36-42 \pm 1$), the patients were re-exposed to budesonide (3×3 mg daily, morning, noon, evening).

For each patient the mean total output per day and per week was determined. The patients measured the weight of the ileostomy bags with a spring balance before emptying and documented the results in a diary. The primary objective of the study was the absolute change of ileostomy output (weight/24 h), comparing phase 1 to week 1 of phase 2, week 1/phase 2 to week 4/phase 2, week 4/phase 2 to phase 3 and phase 1 to phase 3. Body weight and laboratory data were controlled on day 1 (start of phase 1), day 35 (end of phase 2) and day 42 (end of phase 3).

Statistics

The evaluation was performed for the intention-to-treat-population. Differences in mean ileostomy output were analysed by the two-sided Wilcoxon–(Pratt) test. Statistical tests were performed by the program 'Testimate' (version 5.2, IDV – Institut für Datenmanagement und Versuchsplanung, Gauting).

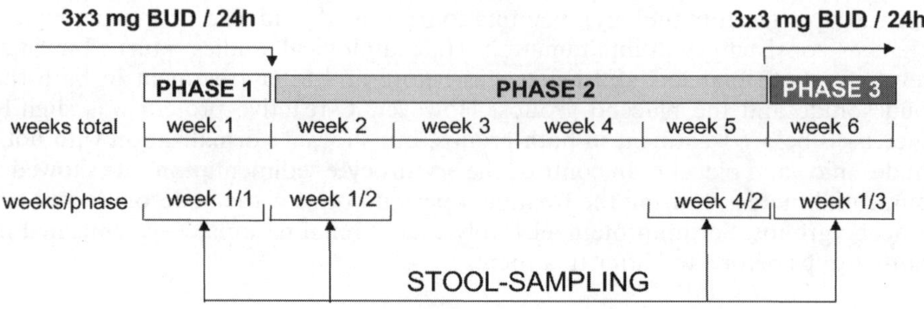

Figure 4   Performance schedule of study 2 (in weeks). BUD = budesonide

Results

The efficacy evaluation was performed for 22 of 23 included patients, because one patient discontinued the study within the first days of phase 1.

Ileostomy output

The ileostomy output after withdrawal of budesonide increased by 295.0 ± 313.0 g (median 188.0 g) from 1195.0 ± 606.9 g to 1490.0 ± 656.4 g daily. This difference was statistically significant ($p < 0.0001$). After re-exposing the patients to budesonide (phase 3), the output decreased by 323.7 ± 322.15 g in comparison to week 4 of phase 2 ($p < 0.0001$). The difference between the ileostomy output of phase 1 and phase 3 (26.9 ± 219.4 g) was not statistically significant ($p = 0.77$) (Figures 5 and 6).

Inflammatory activity

At the commencement of the study, in 11 patients the blood sedimentation rates (ESR_{1h} or ESR_{2h}) were increased, with three patients additionally having increased C-reactive protein (CRP). Whereas for three patients no explanation of these observations could be found, accompanying diseases were assumed responsible in two cases; in two further cases the values had been increased for a longer period of time without known reason. The median of ESR_{1h} did not change between phase 1 and 2, ESR_{2h} and CRP increased slightly during phase 2 and decreased again during phase 3. Clinically relevant abnormalities were found in eight patients for ESR and in five patients for CRP. A clinically relevant deterioration did not occur in any patient for ESR and was observed in two patients for CRP. One of these patients suffered from a relapse of a perianal fistula during the trial; one patient showed an unchanged clinically good status.

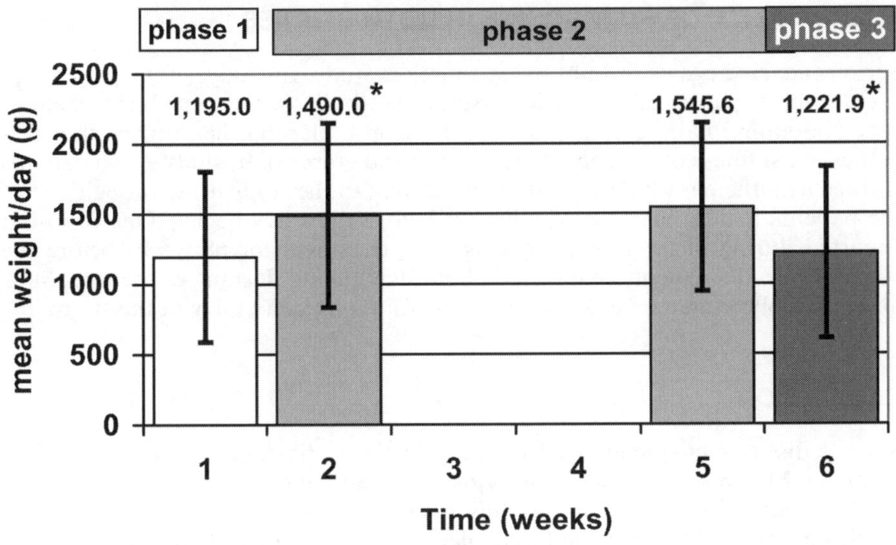

Figure 5 Ileostomy output per day (mean ± standard deviation). Phase 1: treatment with 3×3 mg budesonide (week 1); phase 2: no treatment (week 2–5); phase 3: re-exposure to 3×3 mg budesonide (week 6). *Significant difference ($p < 0.0001$)

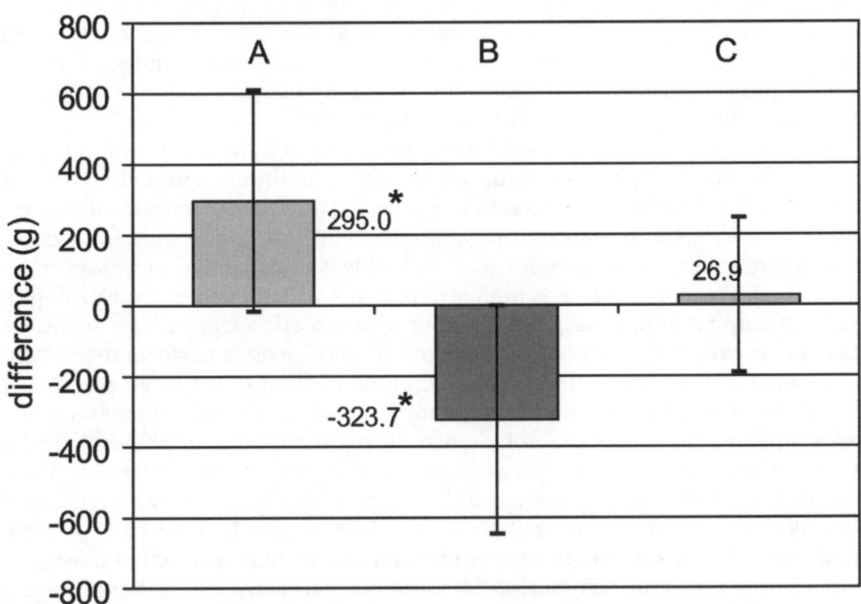

Figure 6 Differences in mean ileostomy output (± standard deviation) per day between study phases. (**A**) Difference week 1 of phase 2–phase 1; (**B**) difference phase 3–week 4 of phase 2; C: difference phase 3–phase 1. *Significant difference ($p < 0.0001$)

TOLERABILITY OF BUDESONIDE IN BOTH STUDIES

Serious adverse events did not occur in either study. In study 1 four patients of each group experienced minor adverse events (budesonide: heartburn, meteorism, abdominal pain, collapse during ileoscopy; placebo: heartburn, skin discolouring, stiffness of interphalangeal joints and cramps). In study 2 two patients showed exanthema, which were possibly related to the study drug, though one of the patients had an increase of bilirubin before the study begins. One drop-out occurred during phase 1. After a long-term treatment for 68 weeks before the study began, the patient complained about itching and flushing of the face, back and arms following the intake of the medication on the first day of the study.

DISCUSSION

Several diseases characterized by chronic watery diarrhoeas, e.g. collagenous colitis and lymphocytic colitis, or cytostatic treatment-induced diarrhoea, have been successfully treated in studies by budesonide[10–14]. These results are confirmed by study 1 presented here, demonstrating an anti-diarrhoeal effect in Crohn's disease patients[9]. This is independent of anti-inflammatory effects and can be explained by influences of corticosteroids on mucosal transport functions[15–18]. As shown by the finding that budesonide was effective in three prednisone-refractory patients, the anti-diarrhoeal effect of corticosteroids may differ[19]. Budesonide is a topically acting corticosteroid that can be applied orally in the form of capsules containing enteric-coated pellets to reach the affected parts of the intestine. Up to 90% of orally administered budesonide is eliminated by a high first-pass effect[20]; therefore the clinically relevant action is restricted to the bowel, reducing the risk of systemic side-effects.

In study 1, based on a double-blind comparison of budesonide and placebo by means of a matched-pair design under hospital conditions with defined diet and controlled fluid intake and schedule, patients showed a decrease of intestinal output of about 400 ml during oral administration of budesonide for 8 days. A clinically relevant decrease in output ($>25\%$) was documented in 60% (12/20) of patients. The response rate was higher in patients with an ileal resection length up to 20 cm compared to those with a higher ileal resection length. This seems to be reasonable, taking into account the ileum's high resorptive performance of about 8.5 L per day in normal subjects and increased ileostomy output in patients with higher resection lengths. The inflammatory activity of the intestine, as shown by endoscopy and histology, did not change during the treatment phase. A decrease in CRP and an increase in ESR were observed in both groups; therefore the two treatment groups remained comparable in terms of inflammatory activity, so that the decrease of ileostomy output secondary to budesonide must be explained by the drug's influence on the transport mechanisms of the intestinal mucosa.

In study 2 the short-term effect demonstrated in study 1 was shown to persist even under long-term conditions. Crohn's disease patients treated for nearly 6 months with 3×3 mg budesonide, for high intestinal output syndrome, showed significantly increased intestinal output upon withdrawal of the drug. After reexposure the output decreased again to the baseline level. This result shows that the efficacy of budesonide on water-absorptive functions of the intestinal mucosa is maintained over several months. The good tolerability of budesonide because of its topical mechanism of action is a further argument to treat patients with high intestinal output syndrome after colectomy with budesonide as long as necessary.

CONCLUSIONS

Topical steroids (budesonide) improve the absorptive capacity of the intestinal mucosa. This functional effect is independent of the anti-inflammatory potency. In the long-term course the effect is strictly and strongly correlated to the administration of the drug.

References

1. Brevinge H, Berglund B, Kock NG. Ileostomy output of gas and feces before and after conversion from conventional to reservoir ileostomy. Dis Colon Rectum. 1992;35:662–9.
2. Tytgat GN, Huibregtse K. Loperamide and ileostomy output – placebo-controlled double-blind study. Br Med J. 1975;2:667.
3. Newton CR. Effect of codeine phosphate, lobomil and isogel on ileostomy function. Gut. 1978;19:377–83.
4. Müller MK, Breuer NF, Goebell H. Behandlung einer chronischen, nicht-sekretorischen Diarrhoe bei Ileostoma mit dem langwirkenden Somatostatinanalog SMS 201-995. Z Gastroenterol. 1988;26:166–8.
5. Neef B, Höring E, von Gaisberg U. Erfolgreiche Behandlung einer lebensbedrohlichen Ileostoma-Diarrhoe mit dem Somatostatin-Analogon Octreotid. Dtsch med Wochenschr. 1994;119:869–74.
6. Herman P, Tan CT, van den Abbeele T et al. Glucocorticosteroids increase sodium transport in the middle ear epithelium. Am J Physiol. 1997;272:C184–90.
7. Bonvalet JP. Regulation of sodium transport by steroid hormones. Kidney Int. 1998;53:49–56.
8. Scheurlen C, Allgayer H, Hardt M, Kruis W. Effect of short-term topical corticosteroid treatment on mucosal enzyme systems in patients with distal inflammatory bowel disease. Hepato-Gastroenterology. 1998;45:1539–45.
9. Ecker KW, Stallmach A, Seitz G, Gierend M, Greinwald R, Achenbach U. Oral budesonide significantly improves water absorption in patients with ileostomy for Crohn disease. Scand J Gastroenterol. 2003;38:288–93.
10. van Gossum A, Schmit A, Peny MO. Oral budesonide for lymphocytic colitis. Am J Gastroenterol. 1998;93:270.
11. Lenfers BHM, Löffler TM, Dröge C et al. Substantial activity of budesonide in patients with irinotecan (CPT-11) and 5-fluorouracil induced diarrhea and failure of loperamide treatment. Ann Oncol. 1999;10:1251–3.
12. Tromm A, Griga T, Möllmann HW, May B, Müller KM, Fisseler-Eckhoff A. Budesonide for the treatment of collagenous colitis: first results of a pilot trial. Am J Gastroenterol. 1999;94:1871–5.
13. Miehlke S, Heymer P, Bethke B et al. Budesonide treatment for collagenous colitis: a randomized, double-blind, placebo-controlled, multicenter trial. Gastroenterology. 2002;123:978–84.
14. Bonderup OK, Hansen JB, Birket-Smith L, Vestergaard V, Teglbjaerg PS, Fallingborg J. Budesonide treatment of collagenous colitis: a randomised, double blind, placebo-controlled trial with morphometric analysis. Gut. 2003;52:248–51.
15. Bastl CP, Schulman G, Cragoe EJ. Low-dose glucocorticoids stimulate electroneutral NaCl absorption in rat colon. Am J Physiol. 1989;257:1027–38.

16. Thiesen A, Tappenden KA, McBurney MI et al. The effect of locally and systemically active steroids on the transport of sugars following intestinal resection in rats is influenced by dietary lipids. Gastroenterology. 1997;112:A910.
17. Coon S, Sundaram U. Mechanism of glucocorticoid mediated reversal of Na:Cl absorption inhibition during chronic ileitis. Gastroenterology. 1999;116:A935 (abstract G4067).
18. Hua A, Weisel S, Sundram U et al. Glucocorticoid mediated reversal of Na:amino acid co-transport inhibition during chronic ileitis. Gastroenterology. 1999;116:A935 (abstract G4069).
19. Lanyi B, Dries V, Dienes HP, Kruis W. Therapy of prednisone-refractory collagenous colitis with budesonide. Int J Colorectal Dis. 1999;14:58–61.
20. Möllmann HW, Hochhaus G, Tromm A et al. Principles of topical versus systemic corticoid treatment in inflammatory bowel disease. In: Möllmann HW, May B, editors. Glucocorticoid Therapy in Chronic Inflammatory Bowel Disease – From Basic Principles to Rational Therapy. Dordrecht: Kluwer, 1996:42–60.

12
Budesonide treatment in pouchitis

A.-J. KROESEN

INTRODUCTION

The pathogenesis of pouchitis is still unknown. In recent years several studies have addressed the epidemiology, pathophysiology, treatment, and dysplasia risk in patients with ulcerative colitis and pouchitis following abdominal colectomy with ileal pouch–anal anastomosis (IPAA); 32% of all patients experienced one or more episodes of pouchitis[1,2].

One of the most common causes of pouchitis is thought to be faecal stasis with an overgrowth of Gram-negative bacteria[3–5]; another hypothesis states that pouchitis results from ischaemia; however, pouchitis seems to be a remanifestation of ulcerative colitis. Inflammatory mediators, cytokines and adhesion molecules and the changes in the terminal ileum confirm this hypothesis[6]. Merrett et al. found a decrease in mucosal permeability[7].

The solution to pouchitis is also the key to ulcerative colitis.

Some interesting facts are known concerning the aetiology of pouchitis. Pouchitis depends on the preoperative extent of ulcerative colitis. Patients with preoperative 'backwash ileitis' are predisposed to chronic pouchitis[8].

Primary sclerosing cholangitis is also a predisposing factor; the cumulative risk of pouchitis after 10 years being 79% vs. 45% for patients without this condition.

As in ulcerative colitis smoking has a positive effect on pouchitis, as stated recently by Merrett et al.[9]. In 1994 Luukkonen and co-workers reported that there is a significant difference in the development of episodic or chronic pouchitis. The cumulative risk of developing chronic pouchitis after 50 months was 0.05 vs. 0.23[2].

Clinical symptoms for pouchitis include anal bleeding, a high white blood count and C-reactive protein, increased stool frequency, incontinence and painful defaecation.

According to the pouchitis disease activity index of the Mayo Clinic, pouchitis severity can be expressed by this score, consisting of endoscopy, histology and clinical symptoms[10].

If pouchitis is suspected pouchoscopy should be performed by histological examination. Medical treatment should be performed only after excluding pelvic sepsis by endosonography or magnetic resonance imaging.

Concerning the medical therapy of pouchitis many substances have been examined, but only a few have reached clinical relevance. Hence only some of those substances will be discussed in the following.

For the medical therapy of pouchitis there are only six placebo-controlled trials and four controlled comparisons. The examined substances are: metronidazole, ciprofloxacin, budesonide, bismuth carbomers, and probiotics.

METRONIDAZOLE AND CIPROFLOXACIN

In two studies by Madden et al. (metronidazole vs. placebo) and Shen et al. (metronidazole vs. ciprofloxacin) a positive effect of metronidazole and ciprofloxacin could be proven. Madden et al. demonstrated a reduction of stool frequency in 73% vs. 9%, and in 55% of the treated patients side-effects were observed[11]. Shen et al. could demonstrate, in seven of nine patients, a significant reduction for both antibiotics, but a greater degree of reduction of the pouchitis disease activity index in the ciprofloxacin group[12].

BUDESONIDE

The most important study concerning pouchitis and budesonide is the study by Sambuelli et al.[13] In a double-blind, double-dummy controlled trial the workers compared budesonide enema vs. metronidazole orally. The budesonide group comprised 12 patients and the metronidazole group 14 patients. The distribution was as follows:

Budesonide:	One × enema (2 mg/100 ml) + two placebo tablets per 6 weeks
Metronidazole:	Two tablets (2 × 500 mg) + one placebo enema per 6 weeks

The pouchitis was defined by the pouchitis disease activity index. The results, as indicated in Figure 1, showed the same effect for budesonide as for metronidazole; however, the incidence of side-effects was 25% in the budesonide group; much less than in the metronidazole group at 57%[13].

CONCLUSIONS

In summary, IPAA is the procedure of choice for patients with ulcerative colitis requiring proctocolectomy, and for many patients with familial adenomatous polyposis. The procedure can be performed safely with predictable complication rates and a high level of patient satisfaction; however, any disorders which may occur need differentiated strategies.

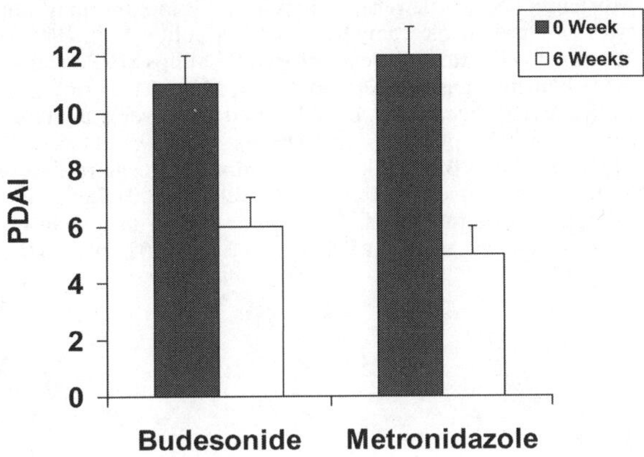

Figure 1 Effect of metronidazole and budesonide on pouchitis disease activity index according to ref. 13

The ileoanal pouch fails in the presence of intractable pouchitis. After excluding peripouchal sepsis this condition should be treated with antibiotics or corticoids.

Uncontrolled fistulas require aggressive surgical treatment to prevent further pelvic sepsis.

In the rare case of a functional failure permanent ileostomy is sometimes the best solution. Complex problems require sophisticated approaches which only specialized centres can offer. Metronidazole is the treatment of choice for pouchitis, and budesonide represents a very good alternative with fewer side-effects.

References

1. Keighley MR. Pouchitis [see comments]. Br J Surg. 1994;81:1091–2.
2. Luukkonen P, Jarvinen H, Tanskanen M, Kahri A. Pouchitis – recurrence of the inflammatory bowel disease? Gut. 1994;35:243–6.
3. McLeod RS, Antonioli D, Cullen J et al. Histologic and microbiologic features of biopsy samples from patients with normal and inflamed pouches. Dis Colon Rectum. 1994;37:26–31.
4. Ruseler-Van Embden JG, Schouten WR, van Lieshout LM. Pouchitis: result of microbial imbalance? Gut. 1994;35:658–64.
5. Ruseler-Van Embden JG, van Lieshout LM, Gosselink MJ, Marteau P. Inability of *Lactobacillus casei* strain GG, *L. acidophilus*, and *Bifidobacterium bifidum* to degrade intestinal mucus glycoproteins. Scand J Gastroenterol. 1995;30:675–80.
6. Evgenikos N, Bartolo DC, Hamer-Hodges DW, Ghosh S. Assessment of ileoanal pouch inflammation by interleukin 1beta and interleukin 8 concentrations in the gut lumen. Dis Colon Rectum. 2002;45:249–55.
7. Merrett MN, Soper N, Mortensen N, Jewell DP. Intestinal permeability in the ileal pouch. Gut. 1996;39:226–30.
8. Schmidt CM, Lazenby AJ, Hendrickson RJ, Sitzmann JV. Preoperative terminal ileal and colonic resection histopathology predicts risk of pouchitis in patients after ileoanal pull-through procedure. Ann Surg. 1998;227:654–62.

9. Merrett MN, Mortensen N, Kettlewell M, Jewell DO. Smoking may prevent pouchitis in patients with restorative proctocolectomy for ulcerative colitis. Gut. 1996;38:362–4.
10. Sandborn WJ, Tremaine WJ, Batts KP, Pemberton JH, Phillips SF. Pouchitis after ileal pouch–anal anastomosis: a Pouchitis Disease Activity Index. Mayo Clin Proc. 1994;69:409–15.
11. Madden MV, McIntyre AS, Nicholls RJ. Double-blind crossover trial of metronidazole versus placebo in chronic unremitting pouchitis. Dig Dis Sci. 1994;39:1193–6.
12. Shen B, Achkar JP, Lashner BA et al. A randomized clinical trial of ciprofloxacin and metronidazole to treat acute pouchitis. Inflamm Bowel Dis. 2001;7:301–5.
13. Sambuelli A, Boerr L, Negreira S et al. Budesonide enema in pouchitis – a double-blind, double-dummy, controlled trial. Aliment Pharmacol Ther. 2002;16:27–34.

13
Chemotherapy-associated diarrhoea

P. REICHARDT

Diarrhoea is a frequent side-effect of chemotherapy regimens containing 5-fluorouracil or irinotecan, occurring in up to 80% of patients. Diarrhoea not only has a detrimental effect on quality of life, it may also limit the dose-intensity of chemotherapy protocols or even prohibit continuation of treatment. Furthermore, approximately 20% of patients treated with 5-fluorouracil and irinotecan experience grade 3 or 4 diarrhoea, which is a potentially life-threatening event.

Chemotherapy-induced diarrhoea is usually an exudative or secretory type of diarrhoea caused by reduced fluid uptake combined with increased secretion and bowel motility.

Treatment options consist of avoiding milk and milk products, alcohol and fat as well as increased oral fluid intake in conjunction with anti-diarrhoeal medication. Standard of care involves synthetic opioids such as loperamide or diphenoxylat. The initial dose of loperamide is 4 mg, followed by 2 mg after every stool. In cases of persistent diarrhoea, the dose should be increased. Patients not responding to high doses of loperamide after 24 h are candidates for octreotid, a long-acting somatostatin analogue. Usual doses range from 100 to 150 µg given subcutaneously three times a day until diarrhoea resolves.

Experimental approaches include the use of the enkephalinase inhibitor acetorphan in combination with loperamide, sucralfate plus nifuroxazid and budesonide, an orally available non-halogenated glucocorticoid with topical anti-inflammatory activity and a high first-pass effect in the liver. Budesonide has been shown to be active in reducing loperamide resistant diarrhoea in irinotecan- and 5-fluorouracil-treated patients.

14
Acute intestinal graft-versus-host disease and budesonide

H. BERTZ

ALLOGENEIC HAEMATOPOIETIC STEM CELL TRANSPLANTATION (alloHSCT)

Introduction

Allogeneic haematopoietic stem cell transplantation (alloHSCT) is the chance for cure in many patients with life-threatening haematopoietic and lymphopoietic malignancies (e.g. acute leukaemia, chronic myeloid leukaemia (CML), aggressive non-Hodgkin's lymphoma and myelodysplastic syndrome (MDS))[1]. Further, alloHSCT has the potential to repopulate the haematopoietic and immunological cell departments in non-malignant, but cell-deficient disorders such as severe aplastic anaemia (SAA) or combined variable immune deficiency syndrome (CIVD).

Major histocompatibility antigen system

In all transplantations (solid organ or HSCT) the major histocompatibility (MHC) antigens are important for transplantation; they play a major role in the physiology of the immune system and are the major barrier for transplantation. In humans the MHC is called HLA and located on chromosome 6. To perform alloHSCT an HLA (human leucocyte antigen)-identical donor is necessary. The HLA system consists of three classes (I, II and III) with many major and minor antigens. In clinical trials it is established that HLA-A and B in class I and HLA-DR and -DQ are relevant for the outcome of alloHSCT[2]. Prior to transplantation the patient and potential donor are tested. Only if the patient/donor pair is identical as regards HLA-A, -B and -DR genes can a safe alloHSCT be performed. The chance of recognition of an identical donor is approximately 30% with siblings and, together with a registered person in the worldwide donor registries, a so-called unrelated donor, nearly 90%. After identification of a matched donor the transplantation is planned, the patient receives a conditioning regimen and the donor is prepared for graft collection.

Graft source

The graft consists of many haematopoietic progenitor cells, the CD34-positive stem cells, out of which the new haematopoietic and immune system may grow. The graft source is the bone marrow (BM) blood of the donor, which is collected by multiple aspirations at the os ileum under general anaesthesia[3]. This BM blood contains a large amount of haematopoietic progenitor cells. Since the development of recombinant haematopoietic growth factors (HGF) such as granulocyte colony-stimulating factor (G-CSF) it is possible to mobilize a sufficient amount of HSC by stimulating the haematopoietic system of the donor using these HGF, and collect them by leukapheresis, the so-called peripheral blood stem cells (PBSC)[4]. The graft consists, besides the progenitor cells, of many immunocompetent lymphocytes; these are necessary to provide the engraftment in the recipient despite the prior conditioning regimen.

Conditioning regimen

The conditioning regimen consists of cytotoxic and lymphotoxic chemotherapy drugs[5] and/or irradiation with three aims: (a) to eliminate the malignant clones, (b) to 'create space' in the pelvis bone for the new graft and (c) to suppress the recipient's immune system to avoid graft rejection. After the conditioning the graft (BM or peripheral blood stem cells) is transfused and the patient experiences a cytopenic phase with the danger of infections and bleeding complications.

T-lymphocyte cells and alloreactivity

Not only the conditioning regimen is able to eliminate the malignant disease, but the transplanted immune system is also able to eradicate the remaining tumour cells, as was shown recently in elderly high-risk patients after a toxicity-reduced intensity-conditioning regimen[6]. The reason is the immune reactivity denoted by the capacity of the immune system to react against non-self antigens (alloreactivity) and self antigens (autoreactivity). T cells play the major role in alloreactivity[7], which is mediated by T cells, B cells and natural killer cells. The T cells carry T-cell receptor-associated adhesion molecules, that bind to monomorphic regions of HLA class I and class II molecules. These are expressed on all cells to different extents.

T cells may be naïve after their development from the new graft, but may also be part of the transplanted graft as activated T cells. For their development and differentiation several cytokines are necessary. The different types of effector cells are: (a) able to kill their target cells directly; (b) able to secret cytokines for further development or (c) to tolerate other cells.

Compared to solid organ transplantation (liver, heart, kidney) in allogeneic haematopoietic stem cell transplantation the achievement of a state of immunological tolerance between the new immunosystem and the recipient's tissue is possible. This will not be achieved in the early months after transplantation, but after tapering the immunosuppression (see below) after 6–12 months. Tolerance depends on many conditions, e.g. HLA disparity, gender of donor and recipient, immunosuppressive prophylaxis or the conditioning regimens.

Graft rejection and graft-versus-leukaemia effect

Special manifestation of the alloreactivity in allogeneic transplantation is the graft rejection, the graft-versus-malignoma/leukaemia (GvM/L) effect and GvHD. In case of graft rejection the recipient's immune system is active, destroying the transplanted graft, because of, e.g. (a) too little conditioning and immunosuppression or (b) a small quantity of the donor's lymphocytes. The graft-versus-malignoma effect (in leukaemias the so-called graft-versus-leukaemia (GvL) effect) is the beneficial side-effect of the alloreaction of the donor lymphoyctes (CTLs and NK cells) against the malignant disease and necessary for achieving long-lasting complete remission.

GvHD

Besides the desired GvL effect GvHD is an outstanding reaction of the donor's immune system against recipient tissue. Acute GvHD (aGvHD) develops in the first 100 days after transplantation as an acute inflammation reaction, mainly of the skin (dermatitis), or mucosa of the mouth (mucositis) with the whole gastrointestinal tract (enteritis) and the liver (hepatitis).

The risk of developing aGvHD also depends on HLA disparity, age and gender of donor and recipient, conditioning regimen or immunosuppressive prophylaxis. Immunosuppressive (IS) prophylaxis for the recipient is necessary to suppress acute GvHD, which is fatal in 100% without prophylaxis[1]. IS consists of either drugs such as cyclosporin, methotrexate, glucocorticoids, mycophenolate-mofetil and tacrolimus and/or T-cell antibodies (anti-CD 52, Mab Campath®) and/or anti-thymocyte/lymphocyte globulins (ATG) (e.g. ATG-S®, Fresenius). Antibodies and ATG are mainly given before transplantation, and the above-mentioned drugs mainly after transplantation. Cyclosporin A (CsA), as an exception, is started shortly before transplantation and is continued intravenously until engraftment and then continued orally; later it is tapered depending on the induction of tolerance.

Risk of aGvHD

The risk of aGvHD increases close to the day of engraftment (leucocytes $>1 \times 10^9$/L) and shortly afterwards, and develops mainly in the first 70 days after transplantation. The degree and area of skin inflammation, the clinical appearance, the level of bilirubin and the quantity of diarrhoea/day are the measures of the severity of aGvHD, and for the overall clinical stage according to organ systems (Table 1).

Pathogenesis of acute intestinal GvHD

Because only a few reports of the upper intestinal tract and aGvHD are published, this overview will deal mainly with GvHD of the gut.

Chronic inflammatory bowel diseases (IBD) show much similarity to acute intestinal GvHD, mainly by the dysbalance of the mucosa-associated immune system and an up-regulation of T-cell activity[9]. For the pathogenesis of GvHD of the gastrointestinal (GI) tract, which plays a major role in the amplification of the systemic disease, endotoxin or lipopolysaccharide (LPS), a constituent of the normal gut flora, are very important[10].

Damage to the gut by the conditioning regimen such as cyclophosphamide or irradiation increases LPS, which promotes the production of tumour necrosis factor alpha (TNF-α), a mediator of intestinal GvHD. The importance of TNF-α in intestinal aGvHD is the same mechanism as described in chronic IBD[11,12]. This is emphasized by studies showing that the severity of the conditioning regimen is responsible for the extent of intestinal GvHD[13]. It is therefore possible to divide the pathophysiology of intestinal GvHD into three phases: (a) conditioning regimen leads to mucosal damage and release of cytokines, e.g. TNF-α; this enhances the expression of MHC antigen on antigen-presenting cells. (b) Donor T cells are attracted and activated. They secrete interleukin 2 (IL-2) and interferon gamma (IFN-γ), which promote further T-cell expansion with cytotoxic T-cell and NK cell responses; the gut mucosa is further damaged. (c) Mononuclear phagocytes are also attracted, and their function is additionally triggered by lipopolysaccharide (LPS) which is now released from the damaged gut mucosa into the blood circulation, stimulating more TNF-α, and again a cytokine storm is started[10].

There are no signs of genetic predisposition, socioeconomic or environmental factors influencing intestinal GvHD, as is shown in IBD, e.g. Crohn's disease (CD)[14,15]. In CD mutations in the NOD2 gene are involved in influencing the immune reaction towards bacterial antigens.

Clinical course of acute intestinal GvHD

The main symptom of intestinal GvHD is diarrhoea, sometimes haemorrhagic and in higher grades associated with cramps. Depending on the volume of the diarrhoea the grade of gut GvHD is defined (Table 1). Sometimes the abdomen is extended and patients experience pain during examination, mainly in the right

Table 1 Extent of organ involvement

	Skin	*Liver*	*Gut*
Stage			
1	Rash <25% of skin	Bilirubin 2–3 mg/dl	Diarrhoea >500 ml/day
2	Rash 25–50% of skin	Bilirubin 3–6 mg/dl	Diarrhoea >1000 ml/day
3	Rash >50 % of skin	Bilirubin 6–15 mg/dl	Diarrhoea >1500 ml/day
4	Generalized erythroderma with bullous formation	Bilirubin >5 mg/dl	Severe abdominal pain with or without ileus
Grade			
I	Stage 1–2	None	None
II	Stage 3 or	Stage 1 or	Stage 1
III	–	Stage 2–3 or	Stage 2–4
IV	Stage 4 or	Stage 4	

Staging and grading of acute GvHD (adapted from ref. 8)

lower part of the abdomen at the ileocaecal region. Bowel movements may be normal, increased or more silent, like an ileus. Considering intestinal GvHD other causes such as infection (e.g. *Clostridium difficile*, cytomegalovirus, herpes simplex virus, rota-virus) or therapy-associated enteritis/mucositis (e.g. neutropenic colitis) should be excluded. Patients with GvHD of the upper GI tract complain of nausea, vomiting, anorexia and pain in the epigastrium.

Diagnostic procedures

The main diagnostic tool is endoscopic examination; this has the advantages of macroscopic assessment of the local mucosa and the possibility of histological confirmation by biopsies. In patients with diarrhoea a sigmoidoscopy is immediately performed. In a case of heavy diarrhoea a total colonoscopy is performed, including the terminal ileum. In a case of vomiting and stomach pain a gastroscopy will be performed.

Recently the evaluation of intestinal aGvHD was studied by high-resolution transabdominal sonography and colour Doppler imaging[16]. Similar procedures have been performed in IBD[17]. Even in patients without clinical symptoms sonographic changes of the gut wall were observed. This non-invasive method is easy to perform, but needs an experienced examiner. Further studies for developing a scoring system are necessary.

Endoscopic evaluation of acute intestinal GvHD

In colonoscopy the macroscopic diagnosis includes: in grade I a nodular-appearing mucosal oedema with a spotted or diffuse erythema, in grade II patchy mucosal bleeding, in grade III an erosive mucosa with aphthoid lesions, and in grade IV ulceration[18]. Similar results could be obtained for the upper GI tract[19].

Histolological pattern of acute intestinal GvHD

The histological pattern includes oedema, active chronic inflammation in the lamina propria with a band of lymphoid or neutrophil cells deep in the lamina propria, lymphocyte inflammation of crypt epithelium with erosive epithelium, erosive epithelium and ulceration by crypt cell destruction and apoptosis[20–22]. In a study by Ponec et al. similar results were obtained for gastric and duodenal GvHD[19]. These histopathological results are mostly obtained when the patient has an overt aGvHD with a high rate of mortality. There is a lack of early inflammatory markers. Activated eosinophils may be such a marker during acute flare-up of GvHD[23]. These have also been shown in IBD[24].

Complications of acute intestinal GvHD

Complications of gut GvHD include loss of water, and loss of proteins including immunoglobulins due to the diarrhoea. The disrupted mucosal barrier is open to the usual intestinal flora consisting of Gram-negative bacteria and yeast pathogens yielding a potential means of entry for bacteria and LPS. The consequences include peritoneal infection, ascites and bacteraemia and fungaemia with sepsis.

These complications are the main cause of the high mortality. Due to the mucosal damage there is a prevalence of bleeding complications in intestinal GvHD. Patients should be observed intensively; platelet count kept above 50×10^6/L; haemostasis equalized and, if necessary, endoscopic manipulation, e.g. laser therapy or cautery, should be performed[25]. In cases of failure of medical therapy (severe bleeding or small-bowel obstruction) surgery can be performed with a successful outcome[26].

Prevention of acute intestinal GvHD

As listed above, many things are done to reduce the incidence and potential severity of GvHD. Patients receive antilymphocyte immunoglobulins (e.g. ATG-S®), lymphocyte antibodies (Mab-Campath®) and immunosuppressive agents (e.g. CsA, methotrexate, mycophenolate mofetil) for GvHD prophylaxis depending on their risk factors for acute GvHD. Several authors have studied how to reduce intestinal GvHD. According to the pathomechanism of acute intestinal GvHD (see section on Clinical course) experimental and clinical studies have shown that gut decontamination for Gram-negative pathogens decreases the incidence and severity of intestinal GvHD[27,28]. Because of the mucosal damage during the pretransplant conditioning regimen enhanced by TNF-α, prophylactic monoclonal antibody (MoAb) neutralizing human TNF-α (MAK 195F) was used to reduce the incidence and severity of intestinal GvHD. This study showed efficient and promising results[29].

Another approach to reduce the mucosal damage caused by pretransplant conditioning is to reduce the intensity and toxicity of the conditioning regimens[30,31]. This has now been confirmed in elderly patients > 60 years of age[32].

Therapy of acute intestinal GvHD

Despite prophylaxis aGvHD occurs frequently and to different extents. Therapy includes the intensification of the above-listed IS therapy (e.g. CsA, monoclonal antibodies, increased doses of systemic glucocorticoids, ATG)[33]. Systemic IS has the disadvantage of increasing the risk of mould and yeast infections and a reduced graft-versus-malignoma effect. The primary treatment, initiation or increase of systemic corticosteroid therapy, may especially lead to severe side-effects such as myopathy, osteoporosis, cataract and increased susceptibility to bacterial and fungal infections.

New therapy strategies to avoid these side-effects have shown efficacy in aGvHD of the GI tract.

TNF-α monoclonal antibody (infliximab)

In CD blocking the activity of TNF-α has shown efficacy[34]. An anti-TNF-α chimaeric monoclonal antibody (infliximab) was used, and its application reduced the fistula[35]. TNF-α is also the key cytokine in the inflammatory cascade of aGvHD. In a recent publication with a small patient group the activity of infliximab to resolve glucocorticoid-refractory aGvHd was proven[36].

Factor XIII

Another similarity between patients with severe aGvHD and CD is a low level of the transglutamine blood coagulation factor XIII, which is necessary for coagulation and wound healing[37]. Supplementation of factor XIII in IBD patients has shown beneficial effects, and also in patients with intestinal GvHD grade IV[38].

Local glucocorticoid therapy

To reduce the systemic IS therapy topical glucocorticoid therapy was used. With beclomethasone dipropionate, a topical corticosteroid administered orally, promising results were reported in treatment of acute intestinal GvHD[39,40].

Besides the oral topical therapy beclomethasone enemas seem to be a potential alternative method for the management of intestinal GvHD[41].

LOCAL THERAPY WITH BUDESONIDE (BUDENOFALK™)

Budenoside capsules (Dr Falk Pharma GmbH, Freiburg, Germany), a topical active glucocorticoid with high affinity to the glucocorticoid receptor[42] and a high anti-inflammatory activity, comprise a preparation releasing budesonide at pH >6.4 which is mainly resorbed in the terminal ileum and ascending colon[43]. The half-life of this preparation is 3.0 h[44]. The systemic bioavailability of budesonide is extremely low[45] due to a rapid first-pass metabolism in the liver[46]. It was used very safely and successfully in chronic IBD (ulcerative colitis[47] and CD[42]). From December 1994 to April 1997 all patients with aGvHD of the GI tract at or above grade II were offered treatment with oral budesonide in addition to a standard increase of systemic IS. The aims of the study were to avoid and/or reduce corticoid side-effects by rapid tapering of the systemic corticosteroid dose and to reach a faster resolution of aGvHD. To show the feasibility of using budesonide in aGvHD we compared the patients in the study with retrospective results in patients receiving only systemic IS.

In Table 2 the endoscopic findings and histology grading are shown according to Kreisel et al.[18]. Not all patients provided complete data.

Resolution of GvHD in the study group (Table 3)

After the diagnosis of acute intestinal GvHD >grade II all patients received systemic IS, mainly increase of corticosteroids (methylprednisolone (MP)) and additionally 3 × 3 mg budesonide (Budenofalk™) orally. Diarrhoea volume and frequency, as well as abdominal pain, were registered. In the case of improvement of the symptoms, decrease of stool frequency and volume, the systemic corticoid dose was rapidly reduced to 50% of the maximum dose, whereas the dosage of budesonide was still maintained. Twenty-two patients received budesonide for a median period of 24 days (range 6–70). Potential side-effects such as nausea or vomiting were not observed in any patient. Only in one patient was a new intestinal pathogen (*Torulopsis glabrata*) found in the stool after initiating oral

Table 2 GvHD grading

	Endoscopic findings (UGI and LGI)	
	Study group (n = 20)	Control group (n = 19)
Grade I/II	10 (50%)	9 (48%)
Grade III	8 (40%)	6 (31%)
Grade IV	2 (10%)	4 (21%)

	Histology grading: (UGI and LGI)	
	Study group (n = 14)	Control group n = (19)
Same as endoscopic	8 (57%)	17 (89%)
One grade difference	4 (29%)	2 (11%)
Two grades difference	2 (14%)	

budenoside. In 17/22 patients (77%) (nine patients with grade II, five patients with grade III and three patients with grade IV) intestinal aGvHD resolved and no relapse occurred. Three patients who did not improve during budesonide therapy had GvHD involvement of other organs and died due to aGvHD with multi-organ failure. Improvement was seen in a median of 12 days (range 3–28) after increasing the glucocorticoid dose and starting the budesonide therapy. The median systemic methylprednisolone dose until improvement or death was 3.8 g (range 1–12 g) and the median budesonide dose was 193 mg (54–725 mg). No relapse of intestinal GvHD occurred after decreasing the methylprednisolone dose while patients were still on budesonide and after cessation of budesonide.

Resolution of GvHD in the control group (Table 3)

In the control group without budesonide intestinal GvHD resolved in 8/19 patients (42%) after intensification of the systemic IS therapy but showed no improvement in 11/19 patients (58%). In 2/8 the acute intestinal GvHD relapsed after tapering the corticosteroid dose. Overall, 13/19 patients (68%) died due to aGvHD. The median dose of systemic methylprednisolone until improvement of intestinal GvHD or death in this group of patients was 4.5 g (1–15 g) and the time prior to improvement in the six patients (32%) who survived was 13 days median (range 7–18). The results are shown in Table 3.

In our survey, despite the fast reduction of glucocorticoids no relapse occurred while budesonide was continued. This was also observed for CD in placebo-controlled studies, showing that low-dose budesonide prolongs time to relapse[48]. Furthermore, our data confirm the importance of endoscopic grading for diagnosis and grading of acute intestinal GvHD, because of the good correlation of endoscopic, histological and clinical classifications of aGvHD in our patients (Table 2)[18].

Table 3 Therapy and outcome

	Study group (n = 22 patients)	Control group (n = 19 patients)	p-Value
Methylprednisolone ↑	20 (90%)	19 (100%)	
Budesonide therapy	22 (100%)	–	
Resolution of aGvHD	17 (77%)	8 (42%)	
Relapse	0	2 (10%)	
Overall response	17 (77%)	6 (32%)	0.01 (significant)
Median days until improvement	12 (3–28)	13 (7–18)	n.s.

Although our study was a non-randomized survey with a retrospective analysis, we conclude that the pH-modified budesonide preparation was very well tolerated in patients with acute intestinal GvHD showing promising results in cases of:

1. Good primary clinical response with budenoside compared to the patients without addition of topical corticosteroids.

2. Safe tapering of the systemic IS was possible without relapse, even in patients with severe GvHD (grade III or IV).

3. In patients who can swallow, budenoside capsules can be applied safely without any side-effects or increase of intestinal infections.

Therefore, early initiation of budesonide therapy should be performed to stop destruction of the intestinal mucosa or to reconstruct the endothelia to avoid bacteraemia or fungaemia.

However, prospective, randomized studies are necessary to prove our results and show whether early extensive reduction of the systemic IS is possible to avoid severe corticoid side-effects. In case of local GvHD of the rectosigmoid application of a budesonide foam should be considered, especially in patients who are unable to swallow[32].

References

1. Hanson JA, Clift RA, Thomas ED et al. Transplantation of marrow from an unrelated donor to a patient with acute leukemia. N Engl J Med. 1980;303:565–7.
2. Ottinger HD, Albert E, Arnold R et al. Consensus on immunogenetic donor search for transplantation of allogeneic bone marrow and peripheral blood stem cells. Bone Marrow Transplant. 1997;20:101–5.
3. Thomas ED, Storb R. Technique for human marrow grafting. Blood. 1970;36:507–15.

4.   Waller CF, Bertz H, Wenger MK et al. Mobilization of peripheral blood progenitor cells for allogeneic transplantation: efficacy and toxicity of a high-dose rhG-CSF regimen. Bone Marrow Transplant. 1996;18:279–83.

5.   Tutschka PJ, Copelan EA, Klein AP. Bone marrow transplantation for leukemia following a new busulfan and cyclophosphamide regimen. Blood. 1987;70:1382–8.

6.   Bertz H, Potthoff K, Finke J. Allogeneic stem cell transplantation from related and unrelated donors in elderly patients with myeloid leukaemia. J Clin Oncol. 2003;21:1480–4.

7.   Kernan NA, Bordignon C, Heller G et al. Graft failure after T-cell depleted human leukocyte antigen identical marrow transplants for leukemia: I. Analysis of risk factors and results of second transplants. Blood. 1989;74:2227–36.

8.   Przepiorka D, Weisdorf D, Martin P et al. Consensus conference on acute GvHD grading. Bone Marrow Transplant. 1995;15:825–8.

9.   Neurath MF, Finotto S, Glimcher LH. The role of Th1/Th2 polarization in mucosal immunity. Nature Med. 2002;8:567–73.

10. Hill GR, Ferrara JLM. The primacy of the gastrointestinal tract as a target organ of acute graft-versus-host disease: rationale for the use of cytokine shields in allogeneic bone marrow transplantation. Blood. 2000;95:2754–9.

11. Plevy SE, Landers CI, Prehn J. A role of TNF-α and mucosal T helper 1 cytokines in the pathogenesis of Crohn's disease. J Immunol. 1997;159:6276–82.

12. Holtmann MH, Gale PR, Neurath MF. Immunotherapeutic approaches in inflammatory bowel diseases. Expert Opin Biol Ther. 2001;1:455–66.

13. Nash A, Pepe MS, Storb R. Acute graft-versus-host disease: analysis of risk factors after allogeneic marrow transplantation and prophylaxis with cyclosporine and methotrexate. Blood. 1992;80:1838.

14. Shanahan F. Crohn's disease. Lancet. 2002;359:62–9.

15. Sandborn WJ, Targan SR. Biological therapy of inflammatory bowel disease. Gastroenterology. 2002;122:1592–608.

16. Klein SA, Martin H, Schreiber-Dietrich D et al. A new approach to evaluating intestinal acute graft-versus-host disease by transabdominal sonography and colour Doppler imaging. Br J Haematol. 2001;115:929–34.

17. Maconi G, Imbesi V, Bianchi Porro G. Doppler ultrasound measurements of intestinal blood flow in inflammatory bowel disease. Scand J Gastroenterol. 1996;31:590–3.

18. Kreisel W, Herbst EW, Schwind B. Endoscopic diagnosis of graft-versus host disease. Eur J Gastroenterol Hepatol. 1994;8:723–9.

19. Ponec RJ, Hackman RC, McDonald GB. Endoscopic and histologic diagnosis of intestinal graft versus-host disease after marrow transplantation Gastrointest Endosc. 1999;49:612–21.

20. Snover DC. Graft versus host disease of the gastrointestinal tract. Am J Surg Pathol. 1990;14(Suppl.1):101–8.

21. Lerner KG, Kao GF, Storb R. Histopathology of graft-vs-host reaction (GvHR) in human recipients of marrow from HLA-matched sibling donors. Transplant Proc. 1974;6:367–71.

22. Carpenter HA, Talley NJ. The importance of clinicopathological correlation in the diagnosis of inflammatory conditions of the colon: histological patterns with clinical implications. Am J Gastroenterol. 2000;95:878–96.

23. Daneshpouy M, Socie G, Lemann M, Rivet J, Gluckman E, Janin A. Activated eosinophils in upper gastrointestinal tract of patients with graft-versus-host disease. Blood. 2002;99:3033–40.

24. Dvorak AM. Ultrastructural evidence for release of major basic protein-containing crystalline cores of eosinophil granules in vitro: cytotoxic potential in Crohn's disease. J Immunol. 1980;125:460–2.

25. Schwartz JM, Wolford JL, Thornquist MD et al. Severe gastrointestinal bleeding after hematopoietic cell transplantation, 1987–1997: incidence, causes, and outcome. Am J Gastroenterol. 2001;96:385–93.

26. Evans J, Percy J, Eckstein R, Ma D, Schnitzler M. Surgery for intestinal graft-versus-host disease: report of two cases. Dis Colon Rectum. 1998;41:1573–6.

27. Moller J, Skirhoj P, Hoiby N, Peterson FB. Protection against graft versus host disease by gut sterilization? Exp Haematol. 1982;10:101.

28. Beelen DW, Elmaagacli A, Muller KD, Hirche H, Schaefer UW. Influence of intestinal bacterial decontamination using metronidazole and ciprofloxacin or ciprofloxacin alone on the development of acute graft-versus-host disease after marrow transplantation in patients

with hematologic malignancies: final results and long term follow-up of an open-label prospective randomized trial. Blood. 1999;93:3267.

29. Holler E, Kolb H-J, Mittermüller J, Kaul J, Ledderose G, Duell T. Modulation of acute graft-versus-host disease after allogeneic bone marrow transplantation by tumour necrosis factor alpha (TNF alpha) release in the course of pretransplant conditioning: role of conditioning regimens and prophylactic application of a monoclonal antibody neutralizing human TNF alpha (MAK 195F). Blood. 1995;86:890–9.

30. Wäsch R, Bertz H, Kunzmann R, Finke J. Incidence of mixed chimerism and clinical outcome in 109 patients after myelo-ablative or reduced conditioning and allogeneic stem cell transplantation. Br J Haematol. 1999;109:743–50.

31. Johansson JE, Brune M, Ekman T. The gut mucosa barrier is preserved during allogeneic, haemopoietic stem cell transplantation with reduced intensity conditioning. Bone Marrow Transplant. 2001;28:737–42.

32. Bertz H, Afting M, Kreisel W, Duffner U, Greinwald R, Finke J. Feasibility and response to budesonide as topical corticosteroid therapy for acute intestinal GvHD. Bone Marrow Transplant. 1999;24:1185–9.

33. Sullivan KM. Graft-vs-host disease. In: Forman SJ, Blume KG, Thomas ED, editors. Bone Marrow Transplantation. Cambridge, MA: Blackwell, 1994:339–46.

34. Baert FJ, D'Haens GR, Peeters M et al. Tumor necrosis factor alpha antibody (infliximab) therapy profoundly down-regulates the inflammation in Crohn's ileocolitis. Gastroenterology. 1999;116:22–8.

35. Present DH, Rutgeerts P, Targan S et al. Infliximab for the treatment of fistulas in patients with Crohn's disease. N Engl J Med. 1999;340:1398–405.

36. Kobbe G, Schneider P, Rohr U et al. Treatment of severe steroid refractory acute graft-versus-host disease with infliximab, a chimeric human/mouse antiTNFalpha antibody. Bone Marrow Transplant. 2001;28:47–9.

37. Pihusch R, Salat C, Gohring P et al. Factor XIII activity levels in patients with allogeneic haematopoietic stem cell transplantation and acute graft-versus-host disease of the gut. Br J Haematol. 2000;117(2):469–76.

38. Grothaus-Pinke B, Gunzelmann S, Fauser AA, Kiehl MG. Factor XIII replacement in stem cell transplant (SCT) recipients with severe graft-versus-host disease of the bowel: report of an initial experience. Transplantation. 2001;72:1456–8.

39. Baehr PH, Levine DS, Bouvier ME et al. Oral beclomethasone dipropionate for treatment of human intestinal graft-versus-host disease. Transplantation. 1995;60:1231–8.

40. McDonald GB, Bouvier ME, Hockenbery DM et al. Oral beclomethasone dipropionate for treatment of intestinal graft-versus-host disease. Gastroenterology. 1998;115:28–35.

41. Wada H, Mori A, Okada M et al. Treatment of intestinal graft-versus-host disease using betamethasone enemas. Transplantation. 2001;72:1451–3.

42. Thomson ABR, Sadowski D, Jenkins R, Wild G. Budesonide in the management of patients with Crohn's disease. Can J Gastroenterol. 1997;11:255–60.

43. Edsbäcker S, Jönsson S, Lindberg C et al. Metabolic pathways of the topical glucocorticoid budesonide in man. Drug Metab Dispos. 1983;6:590–6.

44. Edsbäcker S, Wollmer P, Lindberg C et al. Pharmacokinetics and gastrointestinal transit of budesonide controlled ileal release (CIR) capsules. Gastroenterology. 1993;104(Suppl.):A695.

45. Brogdan RN, McTavish D, Barnes PJ et al. Budesonide. An updated review of its pharmacological properties and therapeutic effects in asthma and rhinitis. Drugs. 1992;44:375–407.

46. Danielson A. Treatment of distal ulcerative colitis with nonsystemic corticosteroid enemas. Scand J Gastroenterol. 1996;31:945–53.

47. Rutgeerts P, Löfberg R, Malchow H. A comparison of budesonide with prednisolone for active Crohn's disease. N Engl J Med. 1994;331:842–5.

48. Löfberg R, Rutgeerts P, Malchow H. Budesonide prolongs time to relapse in ileal and ileocaecal Crohn's disease. A placebo controlled one year study. Gut. 1996;39:82–6.

Section IV
Potential use of budesonide in hepatology

15
Primary biliary cirrhosis

U. LEUSCHNER

Primary biliary cirrhosis (PBC) is a cholestatic as well as an autoimmune liver disease. In contrast to autoimmune hepatitis, glucocorticoids have proved to be ineffective. We suggest that cholestasis possibly reduces the effect of immunosuppressants significantly. Therefore, it could be reasonable first to induce choleresis by using the hypercholeretic bile acid ursodeoxycholic acid (UDCA) and then to initiate immunosuppression by the immunosuppressant budesonide.

The advantage of budesonide in comparison with conventional immunosuppressants is its high relative receptor-binding affinity[1], the low systemic bioavailability of 10–15% and its metabolization to 16α-hydroxyprednisolone and 6β-hydroxybudesonide of which the glucocorticoid activity is one-tenth to one-hundredth that of budesonide. Therefore, with budesonide one could expect a high therapeutic activity with fewer side-effects.

In a 2-year randomized, prospective controlled trial the combination of UDCA (11–15 mg/kg per day) plus budesonide (3×3 mg/day) was compared to UDCA plus placebo[2]. Mainly patients with early stages of the disease were included into the study (Table 1). Combination therapy was significantly superior to UDCA alone concerning liver biochemistry and liver histology (Figures 1 and 2). Serum cortisol levels during and at the end of the study were not suppressed

Table 1 Data of patients treated with UDCA or UDCA/budesonide

	Group A	Group B
No. of patients	20	19
Age (years)	57 ± 2.4	58 ± 2.6
Body weight (kg)	66.4	67.7
Stage of disease:	$3 \times I$	$3 \times I$
	$7 \times II$	$8 \times II$
	$10 \times III$	$8 \times III$

Treatment in group A: 14 mg UDCA/kg/day + 3×3 mg budesonide; in group B: 14 mg/kg/day UDCA + placebo.
Treatment time: 2 years

Modified from ref. 2.

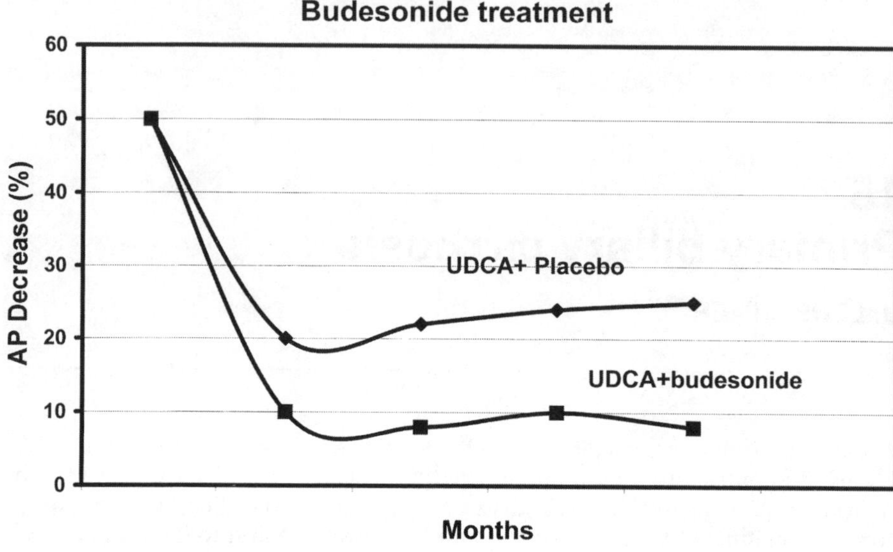

Figure 1 Decrease of AP during UDCA + budesonide vs UDCA + placebo ($p < 0.05$)

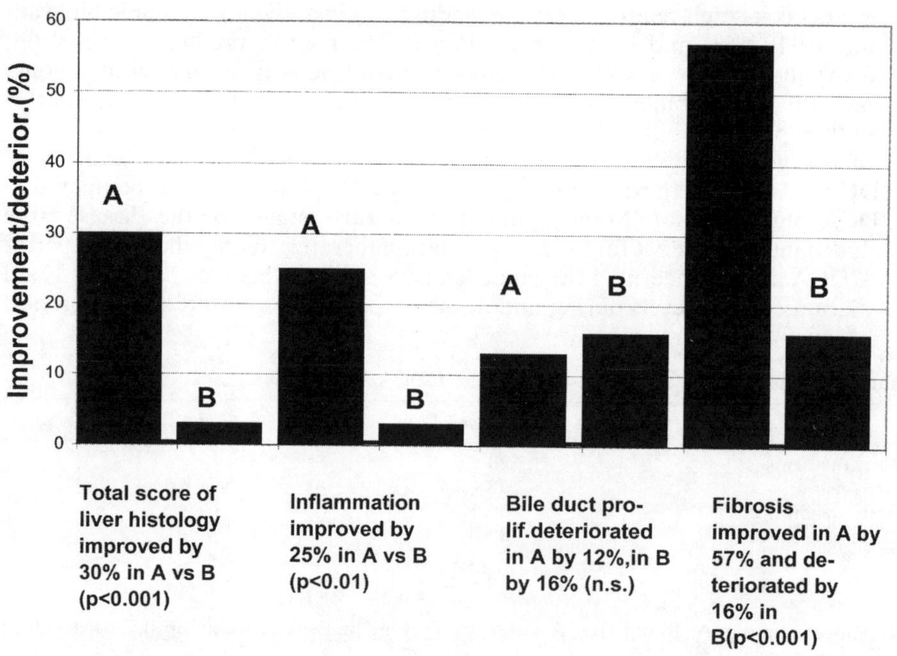

Figure 2 Improvement of histology: group A, UDCA + budesonide; group B, UDCA + placebo

Table 2 Side-effects in patients treated with UDCA/budesonide or UDCA/placebo: UDCA 13 mg/kg/day, budesonide 3 × 3 mg/day (treatment time, 2 years)

Group A (20 patients)	*Group B (19 patients)*
Pretibial oedema: 1. Loss of bone mineral density: 1	Developed oesophageal varices: 2. One of these two experienced haemorrhage. Deterioration of liver function: 1.

Modified from ref. 2.

below the lower reference line by budesonide, and also ACTH-stimulated cortisol secretion before the end of the study was not reduced. Only minor side-effects were observed (Table 2). After treatment ended, the AST, ALT, AP and GLDH serum concentrations increased slightly in the combination group but did not exceed the values of the UDCA group. Therefore, some patients remained on UDCA/budesonide for 3–4 years after the study was completed. In these patients liver values returned to the lower level as observed during the study, and steroid-related side-effects were not detected (unpublished data).

These data were not corroborated by a study from the USA[3]. In this study, however, only patients with a suboptimal response to UDCA were treated, and not naive patients as in our study. Further, the study from the USA was uncontrolled, the patient number was too small and the treatment time too short. Since patients with late stages were also included into this study, the Mayo risk score increased (deterioration of the disease) and bone mass decreased (Table 3), as one could expect before study onset.

These findings cannot be compared with our results of a controlled study, with a larger number of naive patients, with a longer treatment period and mainly with patients in the early stages of the disease. We think that the study from the USA was not conducted with an adequate study design; therefore the conclusions of the authors, that budesonide appears to add minimal, if any, additional benefit to UDCA; that budesonide is associated with a significant worsening of osteoporosis; and that further studies with budesonide are therefore not needed, are at least too rash and cannot be drawn.

Table 3 Oral budesonide in patients with PBC with suboptimal response to ursodeoxycholic acid

Study design	Uncontrolled
Patient number	22
Stage of the disease	Not given*
Treatment time	1 year
Dosage	UDCA 13–15 mg/kg/day; budesonide 9 mg/day
Results	Alkaline phosphatase improved transitory ($p = 0.001$). Mayo score increased ($p = 0.02$). Bone mass decreased ($p < 0.001$)

The authors presume late stages of the disease according to the side-effects observed

From ref. 3

Although it has not yet been shown convincingly that immunosuppression could be helpful in the treatment of PBC, we observed that pregnancy, which represents a time-limited strong immunosuppressive condition, improves liver biochemistry in patients with PBC at the onset of pregnancy and accentuates the effect of UDCA treatment[4]. After delivery liver values return to pre-pregnancy levels. This observation clearly shows that a strong enough immunosuppression could be helpful in the treatment of PBC, which is commonly believed to be resistant to immunosuppressants.

The combination of UDCA with the non-steroidal anti-inflammatory drug Clinoril® (sulindac), which in addition has immunosuppressive properties and in rats increases bile flow 2–3 times[5,6], in PBC patients also improves liver values[7]. Patients who had been treated for 9 years and did not normalize under UDCA alone, showed a statistically significant improvement with the increasing dosage of 100 mg, 200 mg, and in some patients with 300 mg per day when combined with a constant UDCA.

In addition to our previous study[8], and observations of other groups with UDCA/prednisolone or UDCA/prednisolone/azathioprine[9–11], our observations in pregnant women with PBC, and the study with sulindac, strengthen our suggestion that immunosuppressive therapy may be beneficial in combination with UDCA.

SUMMARY AND CONCLUSIONS

Our observations and studies of the literature show that the combination of UDCA with an immunosuppressive drug seems to be superior to UDCA monotherapy in patients in the early stages of PBC. These observations are supported by observations during pregnancy and during the combination of UDCA with the immunosuppressive, anti-inflammatory and choleretic NSAID sulindac. Because of its fewer side-effects than with conventional immunosuppressants we prefer the topical steroid budesonide.

References

1. Möllmann HW, Barth J, Hochhaus G et al. Principles of topical versus systemic corticoid treatment in inflammatory bowel disease. In: Möllmann HW, May B, editors. Glucocorticoid Therapy in Chronic Inflammatory Bowel Disease: From Basic Principles to Rational Therapy. Boston: Kluwer, 1996:42–60.
2. Leuschner M, Maier KP, Schlichting J et al. Oral budesonide and ursodeoxycholic acid for treatment of primary biliary cirrhosis: results of a prospective double-blind trial. Gastroenterology. 1999;117:918–25.
3. Angulo P, Jorgensen RA, Keach JC et al. Oral budesonide in the treatment of patients with primary biliary cirrhosis with a suboptimal response to ursodeoxycholic acid. Hepatology. 2000;31:318–23.
4. Holtmeier J, Leuschner M, Holtmeier W et al. Ursodeoxycholic acid in the treatment of primary biliary cirrhosis (PBC) and primary sclerosing cholangitis (PSC) in pregnancy. Hepatology. 2002;36:491A.
5. Batta AK, Salen G, Pamukcu R et al. Sulindac and its sulfone derivative inhibit colon cancer via modification of intestinal bile acids. Gastroenterology. 1996;110:A490.
6. Bolder U, Trang NV, Hagey LR et al. Sulindac is excreted into bile by a canalicular bile salt pump and undergoes a cholehepatic circulation in rats. Gastroenterology. 1999;117:962–71.

7. Leuschner M, Holtmeier J, Ackermann H et al. The influence of sulindac on patients with primary biliary cirrhosis that responds incompletely to ursodeoxycholic acid: a pilot study. Eur J Gastroenterol Hepatol. 2002;14:1369–76.
8. Leuschner M, Güldütuna S, You T et al. Ursodeoxycholic acid and prednisolone versus ursodeoxycholic acid and placebo in the treatment of early stages of primary biliary cirrhosis. J Hepatol. 1996;25:49–57.
9. Wolfhagen FHJ, van Buuren HR, Schalm SW. Combined treatment with ursodeoxycholic acid and prednisolone in primary biliary cirrhosis. Neth J Med. 1994;44:84–90.
10. Van Buuren HR, Wolfhagen FHJ, Schalm SW. Treatment with ursodeoxycholic acid, as monotherapy and in combination with other agents, in primary biliary cirrhosis. In: Van Berge-Henogouwen GP, van Hoek B, de Groote J et al., editors. Cholestatic Liver Diseases. New Strategies for Prevention and Treatment of Hepatobiliary and Cholestatic Liver Diseases. Dordrecht: Kluwer, 1994:236–45.
11. Wolfhagen FHJ, van Hoogstraten HJF, van Buuren HR et al. Triple therapy with ursodeoxycholic acid, prednisone and azathioprine in primary biliary cirrhosis: a 1-year randomized, placebo-controlled study. J Hepatol. 1998;29:736–42.

16
Autoimmune hepatitis

M. P. MANNS and J. WIEGAND

Autoimmune hepatitis (AIH) is a chronic, mainly periportal hepatitis associated with hypergammaglobulinaemia and circulating autoantibodies. Without treatment the mortality of AIH is up to 90% in 10 years[1,2]. Two fundamental therapeutic goals are important: the induction of remission and the durable maintenance of remission[3]. These goals can be achieved by two different standard treatment schedules including either prednis(ol)one monotherapy or combination therapy with prednis(ol)one and azathioprine. The two therapies are equally effective, but combination therapy is generally preferred because of the marked reduction of side-effects in this group. Many side-effects are related to prednisone, depending upon the steroid dose. Thus, the administration of azathioprine offers the opportunity to avoid or reduce steroids. A second attractive option is to replace prednisone by steroids with potentially fewer systemic side-effects.

Budesonide is a synthetic glucocorticoid which is derived from 16α-hydroxyprednisolone. Its affinity to the glucocorticoid receptor is about 15 times higher than that of prednisolone. Budesonide undergoes a high first-pass metabolism in the liver, which reduces its systemic bioavailability to 10%. It is a common drug for allergic pulmonary disease and inflammatory bowel disease. So far, there have been several small studies which have evaluated its efficacy in the case of autoimmune hepatitis.

In a study treating 13 AIH patients with initially 6–8 mg of budesonide daily over a period of 9 months budesonide decreased aminotransferase levels to normal limits and was well tolerated[4]. No patient experienced subjective corticosteroid side-effects or more marked signs of cushingoid habitus during the trial period. Cirrhotic patients experienced a significantly stronger decrease of plasma cortisol than non-cirrhotic patients, but the mean reference value remained above the lowest reference value.

In a single case with recurrence of AIH type II after liver transplantation the initial high-dose prednisone therapy was replaced by 2×3 mg budesonide per day plus a low maintenance therapy of 2.5 mg prednisone due to appearance of cushingoid symptoms. After the treatment had changed the cushingoid side-effects disappeared and aminotransferase levels normalized within 5 months.

A later study from our department treated nine patients with 2×3 up to 2×5 mg budesonide per day for 1 year[5]. Three patients were additionally treated with

100 mg azathioprine; four patients reached a complete remission and three patients an incomplete remission. Histological improvement could be observed in two patients while one patient remained unchanged and four patients showed progressive disease. In our experience side-effects could be managed with dose reduction, or improved after decrease of hepatic inflammation. Thus, in cases with AIH and severe inflammation or cirrhosis budesonide is metabolized to a lower degree. A possible explanation is the reduced liver function and the occurrence of portosystemic shunts. Metabolism and side-effects improve during decrease of inflammation, or the improvement of liver function.

The results of these trials indicate that remission of AIH can be achieved when prednisolone is replaced by budesonide. However, the main advantage of budesonide for future treatment of AIH is to replace prednisolone in long-term maintenance therapy to reduce steroid side-effects. This potential benefit has not been prospectively proven so far.

The change to budesonide in 10 patients on an immunosuppressive maintenance therapy was associated with a low frequency of remission, occurrence of treatment failure, and side-effects[6].

Therefore, further studies have to evaluate the safety, efficacy and tolerance of budesonide in maintenance therapy of AIH. Long-term results of patients initially treated with budesonide monotherapy or with budesonide and azathioprine are still pending.

References

1.   Geall MG, Schoenfield LJ, Summerskill WHJ. Classification and treatment of chronic active liver disease. Gastroenterology. 1968;55:724–9.
2.   Soloway RD, Summerskill WHJ, Baggenstoss AH et al. Clinical, biochemical and histologic remission of severe chronic active liver disease: a controlled study of treatments and early prognosis. Gastroenterology. 1972;63:820–33.
3.   Manns MP, Strassburg CP. Autoimme hepatitis: clinical challenges. Gastroenterology. 2001; 120:1502–17.
4.   Danielsson A, Prytz H. Oral budesonide for treatment of autoimmune chronic active hepatitis. Aliment Pharmacol Ther. 1994;8:585–90.
5.   Schüler A, Möllmann HW, Manns MP. Treatment of autoimmune hepatitis with budesonide. Hepatology. 1995;22:488A.
6.   Czaja AJ, Lindor KD. Failure of budesonide in a pilot study of treatment-dependent autoimmune hepatitis. Gastroenterology. 2000;119:1312–16.

Index

Falk Symposium Series

43. Reutter W, Popper H, Arias IM, Heinrich PC, Keppler D, Landmann L, eds.: *Modulation of Liver Cell Expression*. Falk Symposium No. 43. 1987   ISBN: 0-85200-677-2*

44. Boyer JL, Bianchi L, eds.: *Liver Cirrhosis*. Falk Symposium No. 44. 1987
ISBN: 0-85200-993-3*

45. Paumgartner G, Stiehl A, Gerok W, eds.: *Bile Acids and the Liver*. Falk Symposium No. 45. 1987   ISBN: 0-85200-675-6*

46. Goebell H, Peskar BM, Malchow H, eds.: *Inflammatory Bowel Diseases – Basic Research & Clinical Implications*. Falk Symposium No. 46. 1988   ISBN: 0-7462-0067-6*

47. Bianchi L, Holt P, James OFW, Butler RN, eds.: *Aging in Liver and Gastrointestinal Tract*. Falk Symposium No. 47. 1988   ISBN: 0-7462-0066-8*

48. Heilmann C, ed.: *Calcium-Dependent Processes in the Liver*. Falk Symposium No. 48. 1988   ISBN: 0-7462-0075-7*

50. Singer MV, Goebell H, eds.: *Nerves and the Gastrointestinal Tract*. Falk Symposium No. 50. 1989   ISBN: 0-7462-0114-1

51. Bannasch P, Keppler D, Weber G, eds.: *Liver Cell Carcinoma*. Falk Symposium No. 51. 1989   ISBN: 0-7462-0111-7

52. Paumgartner G, Stiehl A, Gerok W, eds.: *Trends in Bile Acid Research*. Falk Symposium No. 52. 1989   ISBN: 0-7462-0112-5

53. Paumgartner G, Stiehl A, Barbara L, Roda E, eds.: *Strategies for the Treatment of Hepatobiliary Diseases*. Falk Symposium No. 53. 1990   ISBN: 0-7923-8903-4

54. Bianchi L, Gerok W, Maier K-P, Deinhardt F, eds.: *Infectious Diseases of the Liver*. Falk Symposium No. 54. 1990   ISBN: 0-7923-8902-6

55. Falk Symposium No. 55 not published

55B. Hadziselimovic F, Herzog B, Bürgin-Wolff A, eds.: *Inflammatory Bowel Disease and Coeliac Disease in Children*. International Falk Symposium. 1990 ISBN 0-7462-0125-7

56. Williams CN, eds.: *Trends in Inflammatory Bowel Disease Therapy*. Falk Symposium No. 56. 1990   ISBN: 0-7923-8952-2

57. Bock KW, Gerok W, Matern S, Schmid R, eds.: *Hepatic Metabolism and Disposition of Endo- and Xenobiotics*. Falk Symposium No. 57. 1991   ISBN: 0-7923-8953-0

58. Paumgartner G, Stiehl A, Gerok W, eds.: *Bile Acids as Therapeutic Agents: From Basic Science to Clinical Practice*. Falk Symposium No. 58. 1991   ISBN: 0-7923-8954-9

59. Halter F, Garner A, Tytgat GNJ, eds.: *Mechanisms of Peptic Ulcer Healing*. Falk Symposium No. 59. 1991   ISBN: 0-7923-8955-7

60. Goebell H, Ewe K, Malchow H, Koelbel Ch, eds.: *Inflammatory Bowel Diseases – Progress in Basic Research and Clinical Implications*. Falk Symposium No. 60. 1991
ISBN: 0-7923-8956-5

61. Falk Symposium No. 61 not published

62. Dowling RH, Folsch UR, Löser Ch, eds.: *Polyamines in the Gastrointestinal Tract*. Falk Symposium No. 62. 1992   ISBN: 0-7923-8976-X

63. Lentze MJ, Reichen J, eds.: *Paediatric Cholestasis: Novel Approaches to Treatment*. Falk Symposium No. 63. 1992   ISBN: 0-7923-8977-8

64. Demling L, Frühmorgen P, eds.: *Non-Neoplastic Diseases of the Anorectum*. Falk Symposium No. 64. 1992   ISBN: 0-7923-8979-4

64B. Gressner AM, Ramadori G, eds.: *Molecular and Cell Biology of Liver Fibrogenesis*. International Falk Symposium. 1992   ISBN: 0-7923-8980-8

*These titles were published under the MTP Press imprint.

Falk Symposium Series

65. Hadziselimovic F, Herzog B, eds.: *Inflammatory Bowel Diseases and Morbus Hirschprung*. Falk Symposium No. 65. 1992 ISBN: 0-7923-8995-6

66. Martin F, McLeod RS, Sutherland LR, Williams CN, eds.: *Trends in Inflammatory Bowel Disease Therapy*. Falk Symposium No. 66. 1993 ISBN: 0-7923-8827-5

67. Schölmerich J, Kruis W, Goebell H, Hohenberger W, Gross V, eds.: *Inflammatory Bowel Diseases – Pathophysiology as Basis of Treatment*. Falk Symposium No. 67. 1993
ISBN: 0-7923-8996-4

68. Paumgartner G, Stiehl A, Gerok W, eds.: *Bile Acids and The Hepatobiliary System: From Basic Science to Clinical Practice*. Falk Symposium No. 68. 1993
ISBN: 0-7923-8829-1

69. Schmid R, Bianchi L, Gerok W, Maier K-P, eds.: *Extrahepatic Manifestations in Liver Diseases*. Falk Symposium No. 69. 1993 ISBN: 0-7923-8821-6

70. Meyer zum Büschenfelde K-H, Hoofnagle J, Manns M, eds.: *Immunology and Liver*. Falk Symposium No. 70. 1993 ISBN: 0-7923-8830-5

71. Surrenti C, Casini A, Milani S, Pinzani M , eds.: *Fat-Storing Cells and Liver Fibrosis*. Falk Symposium No. 71. 1994 ISBN: 0-7923-8842-9

72. Rachmilewitz D, ed.: *Inflammatory Bowel Diseases – 1994*. Falk Symposium No. 72. 1994 ISBN: 0-7923-8845-3

73. Binder HJ, Cummings J, Soergel KH, eds.: *Short Chain Fatty Acids*. Falk Symposium No. 73. 1994 ISBN: 0-7923-8849-6

73B.Möllmann HW, May B, eds.: *Glucocorticoid Therapy in Chronic Inflammatory Bowel Disease: from basic principles to rational therapy*. International Falk Workshop. 1996
ISBN 0-7923-8708-2

74. Keppler D, Jungermann K, eds.: *Transport in the Liver*. Falk Symposium No. 74. 1994
ISBN: 0-7923-8858-5

74B.Stange EF, ed.: *Chronic Inflammatory Bowel Disease*. Falk Symposium. 1995
ISBN: 0-7923-8876-3

75. van Berge Henegouwen GP, van Hoek B, De Groote J, Matern S, Stockbrügger RW, eds.: *Cholestatic Liver Diseases: New Strategies for Prevention and Treatment of Hepatobiliary and Cholestatic Liver Diseases*. Falk Symposium 75. 1994.
ISBN: 0-7923-8867-4

76. Monteiro E, Tavarela Veloso F, eds.: *Inflammatory Bowel Diseases: New Insights into Mechanisms of Inflammation and Challenges in Diagnosis and Treatment*. Falk Symposium 76. 1995. ISBN 0-7923-8884-4

77. Singer MV, Ziegler R, Rohr G, eds.: *Gastrointestinal Tract and Endocrine System*. Falk Symposium 77. 1995. ISBN 0-7923-8877-1

78. Decker K, Gerok W, Andus T, Gross V, eds.: *Cytokines and the Liver*. Falk Symposium 78. 1995. ISBN 0-7923-8878-X

79. Holstege A, Schölmerich J, Hahn EG, eds.: *Portal Hypertension*. Falk Symposium 79. 1995. ISBN 0-7923-8879-8

80. Hofmann AF, Paumgartner G, Stiehl A, eds.: *Bile Acids in Gastroenterology: Basic and Clinical Aspects*. Falk Symposium 80. 1995 ISBN 0-7923-8880-1

81. Riecken EO, Stallmach A, Zeitz M, Heise W, eds.: *Malignancy and Chronic Inflammation in the Gastrointestinal Tract – New Concepts*. Falk Symposium 81. 1995
ISBN 0-7923-8889-5

82. Fleig WE, ed.: *Inflammatory Bowel Diseases: New Developments and Standards*. Falk Symposium 82. 1995 ISBN 0-7923-8890-6

82B. Paumgartner G, Beuers U, eds.: *Bile Acids in Liver Diseases.* International Falk Workshop. 1995   ISBN 0-7923-8891-7

83. Dobrilla G, Felder M, de Pretis G, eds.: *Advances in Hepatobiliary and Pancreatic Diseases: Special Clinical Topics.* Falk Symposium 83. 1995.   ISBN 0-7923-8892-5

84. Fromm H, Leuschner U, eds.: *Bile Acids – Cholestasis – Gallstones: Advances in Basic and Clinical Bile Acid Research.* Falk Symposium 84. 1995   ISBN 0-7923-8893-3

85. Tytgat GNJ, Bartelsman JFWM, van Deventer SJH, eds.: *Inflammatory Bowel Diseases.* Falk Symposium 85. 1995   ISBN 0-7923-8894-1

86. Berg PA, Leuschner U, eds.: *Bile Acids and Immunology.* Falk Symposium 86. 1996   ISBN 0-7923-8700-7

87. Schmid R, Bianchi L, Blum HE, Gerok W, Maier KP, Stalder GA, eds.: *Acute and Chronic Liver Diseases: Molecular Biology and Clinics.* Falk Symposium 87. 1996   ISBN 0-7923-8701-5

88. Blum HE, Wu GY, Wu CH, eds.: *Molecular Diagnosis and Gene Therapy.* Falk Symposium 88. 1996   ISBN 0-7923-8702-3

88B. Poupon RE, Reichen J, eds.: *Surrogate Markers to Assess Efficacy of TReatment in Chronic Liver Diseases.* International Falk Workshop. 1996   ISBN 0-7923-8705-8

89. Reyes HB, Leuschner U, Arias IM, eds.: *Pregnancy, Sex Hormones and the Liver.* Falk Symposium 89. 1996   ISBN 0-7923-8704-X

89B. Broelsch CE, Burdelski M, Rogiers X, eds.: *Cholestatic Liver Diseases in Children and Adults.* International Falk Workshop. 1996   ISBN 0-7923-8710-4

90. Lam S-K, Paumgartner P, Wang B, eds.: *Update on Hepatobiliary Diseases 1996.* Falk Symposium 90. 1996   ISBN 0-7923-8715-5

91. Hadziselimovic F, Herzog B, eds.: *Inflammatory Bowel Diseases and Chronic Recurrent Abdominal Pain.* Falk Symposium 91. 1996   ISBN 0-7923-8722-8

91B. Alvaro D, Benedetti A, Strazzabosco M, eds.: *Vanishing Bile Duct Syndrome – Pathophysiology and Treatment.* International Falk Workshop. 1996   ISBN 0-7923-8721-X

92. Gerok W, Loginov AS, Pokrowskij VI, eds.: *New Trends in Hepatology 1996.* Falk Symposium 92. 1997   ISBN 0-7923-8723-6

93. Paumgartner G, Stiehl A, Gerok W, eds.: *Bile Acids in Hepatobiliary Diseases – Basic Research and Clinical Application.* Falk Symposium 93. 1997   ISBN 0-7923-8725-2

94. Halter F, Winton D, Wright NA, eds.: *The Gut as a Model in Cell and Molecular Biology.* Falk Symposium 94. 1997   ISBN 0-7923-8726-0

94B. Kruse-Jarres JD, Schölmerich J, eds.: *Zinc and Diseases of the Digestive Tract.* International Falk Workshop. 1997   ISBN 0-7923-8724-4

95. Ewe K, Eckardt VF, Enck P, eds.: *Constipation and Anorectal Insufficiency.* Falk Symposium 95. 1997   ISBN 0-7923-8727-9

96. Andus T, Goebell H, Layer P, Schölmerich J, eds.: *Inflammatory Bowel Disease – from Bench to Bedside.* Falk Symposium 96. 1997   ISBN 0-7923-8728-7

97. Campieri M, Bianchi-Porro G, Fiocchi C, Schölmerich J, eds. *Clinical Challenges in Inflammatory Bowel Diseases: Diagnosis, Prognosis and Treatment.* Falk Symposium 97. 1998   ISBN 0-7923-8733-3

98. Lembcke B, Kruis W, Sartor RB, eds. *Systemic Manifestations of IBD: The Pending Challenge for Subtle Diagnosis and Treatment.* Falk Symposium 98. 1998   ISBN 0-7923-8734-1

99. Goebell H, Holtmann G, Talley NJ, eds. *Functional Dyspepsia and Irritable Bowel Syndrome: Concepts and Controversies.* Falk Symposium 99. 1998
ISBN 0-7923-8735-X

100. Blum HE, Bode Ch, Bode JCh, Sartor RB, eds. *Gut and the Liver.* Falk Symposium 100. 1998
ISBN 0-7923-8736-8

101. Rachmilewitz D, ed. *V International Symposium on Inflammatory Bowel Diseases.* Falk Symposium 101. 1998
ISBN 0-7923-8743-0

102. Manns MP, Boyer JL, Jansen PLM, Reichen J, eds. *Cholestatic Liver Diseases.* Falk Symposium 102. 1998
ISBN 0-7923-8746-5

102B. Manns MP, Chapman RW, Stiehl A, Wiesner R, eds. *Primary Sclerosing Cholangitis.* International Falk Workshop. 1998.
ISBN 0-7923-8745-7

103. Häussinger D, Jungermann K, eds. *Liver and Nervous System.* Falk Symposium 102. 1998
ISBN 0-7924-8742-2

103B. Häussinger D, Heinrich PC, eds. *Signalling in the Liver.* International Falk Workshop. 1998
ISBN 0-7923-8744-9

103C. Fleig W, ed. *Normal and Malignant Liver Cell Growth.* International Falk Workshop. 1998
ISBN 0-7923-8748-1

104. Stallmach A, Zeitz M, Strober W, MacDonald TT, Lochs H, eds. *Induction and Modulation of Gastrointestinal Inflammation.* Falk Symposium 104. 1998
ISBN 0-7923-8747-3

105. Emmrich J, Liebe S, Stange EF, eds. *Innovative Concepts in Inflammatory Bowel Diseases.* Falk Symposium 105. 1999
ISBN 0-7923-8749-X

106. Rutgeerts P, Colombel J-F, Hanauer SB, Schölmerich J, Tytgat GNJ, van Gossum A, eds. *Advances in Inflammatory Bowel Diseases.* Falk Symposium 106. 1999
ISBN 0-7923-8750-3

107. Špičák J, Boyer J, Gilat T, Kotrlik K, Mareček Z, Paumgartner G, eds. *Diseases of the Liver and the Bile Ducts – New Aspects and Clinical Implications.* Falk Symposium 107. 1999
ISBN 0-7923-8751-1

108. Paumgartner G, Stiehl A, Gerok W, Keppler D, Leuschner U, eds. *Bile Acids and Cholestasis.* Falk Symposium 108. 1999
ISBN 0-7923-8752-X

109. Schmiegel W, Schölmerich J, eds. *Colorectal Cancer – Molecular Mechanisms, Premalignant State and its Prevention.* Falk Symposium 109. 1999
ISBN 0-7923-8753-8

110. Domschke W, Stoll R, Brasitus TA, Kagnoff MF, eds. *Intestinal Mucosa and its Diseases – Pathophysiology and Clinics.* Falk Symposium 110. 1999
ISBN 0-7923-8754-6

110B. Northfield TC, Ahmed HA, Jazwari RP, Zentler-Munro PL, eds. *Bile Acids in Hepatobiliary Disease.* Falk Workshop. 2000
ISBN 0-7923-8755-4

111. Rogler G, Kullmann F, Rutgeerts P, Sartor RB, Schölmerich J, eds. *IBD at the End of its First Century.* Falk Symposium 111. 2000
ISBN 0-7923-8756-2

112. Krammer HJ, Singer MV, eds. *Neurogastroenterology: From the Basics to the Clinics.* Falk Symposium 112. 2000
ISBN 0-7923-8757-0

113. Andus T, Rogler G, Schlottmann K, Frick E, Adler G, Schmiegel W, Zeitz M, Schölmerich J, eds. *Cytokines and Cell Homeostasis in the Gastrointestinal Tract.* Falk Symposium 113. 2000
ISBN 0-7923-8758-9

114. Manns MP, Paumgartner G, Leuschner U, eds. *Immunology and Liver.* Falk Symposium 114. 2000
ISBN 0-7923-8759-7

Falk Symposium Series

115. Boyer JL, Blum HE, Maier K-P, Sauerbruch T, Stalder GA, eds. *Liver Cirrhosis and its Development*. Falk Symposium 115. 2000   ISBN 0-7923-8760-0

116. Riemann JF, Neuhaus H, eds. *Interventional Endoscopy in Hepatology*. Falk Symposium 116. 2000   ISBN 0-7923-8761-9

116A. Dienes HP, Schirmacher P, Brechot C, Okuda K, eds. *Chronic Hepatitis: New Concepts of Pathogenesis, Diagnosis and Treatment*. Falk Workshop. 2000
     ISBN 0-7923-8763-5

117. Gerbes AL, Beuers U, Jüngst D, Pape GR, Sackmann M, Sauerbruch T, eds. *Hepatology 2000 – Symposium in Honour of Gustav Paumgartner*. Falk Symposium 117. 2000
     ISBN 0-7923-8765-1

117A. Acalovschi M, Paumgartner G, eds. *Hepatobiliary Diseases: Cholestasis and Gallstones*. Falk Workshop. 2000   ISBN 0-7923-8770-8

118. Frühmorgen P, Bruch H-P, eds. *Non-Neoplastic Diseases of the Anorectum*. Falk Symposium 118. 2001   ISBN 0-7923-8766-X

119. Fellermann K, Jewell DP, Sandborn WJ, Schölmerich J, Stange EF, eds. *Immunosuppression in Inflammatory Bowel Diseases – Standards, New Developments, Future Trends*. Falk Symposium 119. 2001   ISBN 0-7923-8767-8

120. van Berge Henegouwen GP, Keppler D, Leuschner U, Paumgartner G, Stiehl A, eds. *Biology of Bile Acids in Health and Disease*. Falk Symposium 120. 2001
     ISBN 0-7923-8768-6

121. Leuschner U, James OFW, Dancygier H, eds. *Steatohepatitis (NASH and ASH)*. Falk Symposium 121. 2001   ISBN 0-7923-8769-4

121A. Matern S, Boyer JL, Keppler D, Meier-Abt PJ, eds. *Hepatobiliary Transport: From Bench to Bedside*. Falk Workshop. 2001   ISBN 0-7923-8771-6

122. Campieri M, Fiocchi C, Hanauer SB, Jewell DP, Rachmilewitz R, Schölmerich J, eds. *Inflammatory Bowel Disease – A Clinical Case Approach to Pathophysiology, Diagnosis, and Treatment*. Falk Symposium 122. 2002   ISBN 0-7923-8772-4

123. Rachmilewitz D, Modigliani R, Podolsky DK, Sachar DB, Tozun N, eds. *VI International Symposium on Inflammatory Bowel Diseases*. Falk Symposium 123. 2002
     ISBN 0-7923-8773-2

124. Hagenmüller F, Manns MP, Musmann H-G, Riemann JF, eds. *Medical Imaging in Gastroenterology and Hepatology*. Falk Symposium 124. 2002   ISBN 0-7923-8774-0

125. Gressner AM, Heinrich PC, Matern S, eds. *Cytokines in Liver Injury and Repair*. Falk Symposium 125. 2002   ISBN 0-7923-8775-9

126. Gupta S, Jansen PLM, Klempnauer J, Manns MP, eds. *Hepatocyte Transplantation*. Falk Symposium 126. 2002   ISBN 0-7923-8776-7

127. Hadziselimovic F, ed. *Autoimmune Diseases in Paediatric Gastroenterology*. Falk Symposium 127. 2002   ISBN 0-7923-8778-3

127A. Berr F, Bruix J, Hauss J, Wands J, Wittekind Ch, eds. *Malignant Liver Tumours: Basic Concepts and Clinical Management*. Falk Workshop. 2002   ISBN 0-7923-8779-1

128. Scheppach W, Scheurlen M, eds. *Exogenous Factors in Colonic Carcinogenesis*. Falk Symposium 128. 2002   ISBN 0-7923-8780-5

129. Paumgartner G, Keppler D, Leuschner U, Stiehl A, eds. *Bile Acids: From Genomics to Disease and Therapy*. Falk Symposium 129. 2002   ISBN 0-7923-8781-3

129A. Leuschner U, Berg PA, Holtmeier J, eds. *Bile Acids and Pregnancy*. Falk Workshop. 2002   ISBN 0-7923-8782-1

Falk Symposium Series

130. Holtmann G, Talley NJ, eds. *Gastrointestinal Inflammation and Disturbed Gut Function: The Challenge of New Concepts.* Falk Symposium 130. 2003
ISBN 0-7923-8783-X

131. Herfarth H, Feagan BJ, Folsch UR, Schölmerich J, Vatn MH, Zeitz M, eds. *Targets of Treatment in Chronic Inflammatory Bowel Diseases.* Falk Symposium 131. 2003
ISBN 0-7923-8784-8

132. Galle PR, Gerken G, Schmidt WE, Wiedenmann B, eds. *Disease Progression and Carcinogenesis in the Gastrointestinal Tract.* Falk Symposium 132. 2003
ISBN 0-7923-8785-6

132A. Staritz M, Adler G, Knuth A, Schmiegel W, Schmoll H-J, eds. *Side-effects of Chemotherapy on the Gastrointestinal Tract.* Falk Workshop. 2003
ISBN 0-7923-8791-0

132B. Reutter W, Schuppan D, Tauber R, Zeitz M, eds. *Cell Adhesion Molecules in Health and Disease.* Falk Workshop. 2003
ISBN 0-7923-8786-4

133. Duchmann R, Blumberg R, Neurath M, Schölmerich J, Strober W, Zeitz M. *Mechanisms of Intestinal Inflammation: Implications for Therapeutic Intervention in IBD.* Falk Symposium 133. 2004
ISBN 0-7923-8787-2

134. Dignass A, Lochs H, Stange E. *Trends and Controversies in IBD – Evidence-Based Approach or Individual Management?* Falk Symposium 134. 2004
ISBN 0-7923-8788-0

134A. Dignass A, Gross HJ, Buhr V, James OFW. *Topical Steroids in Gastroenterology and Hepatology.* Falk Workshop. 2004
ISBN 0-7923-8789-9